Coronary CT Angiography

Marc Dewey

Coronary CT Angiography

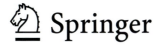

Privatdozent Dr. med. Marc Dewey
Charité - Universitätsmedizin Berlin
Humboldt-Universität zu Berlin
Freie Universität Berlin
Institut für Radiologie
Charitéplatz 1
10117 Berlin
Germany
marc.dewey@charite.de

ISBN 978-3-540-79843-9   e-ISBN 978-3-540-79844-6

DOI: 10.1007/978-3-540-79844-6

Library of Congress Control Number: 2008926106

© 2009 Springer-Verlag Berlin Heidelberg

This work is subject to copyright. All rights are reserved, whether the whole or part of the material is concerned, specifically the rights of translation, reprinting, reuse of illustrations, recitation, broadcasting, reproduction on microfilm or in any other way, and storage in data banks. Duplication of this publication or parts thereof is permitted only under the provisions of the German Copyright Law of September 9, 1965, in its current version, and permission for use must always be obtained from Springer. Violations are liable to prosecution under the German Copyright Law.

The use of general descriptive names, registered names, trademarks, etc. in this publication does not imply, even in the absence of a specific statement, that such names are exempt from the relevant protective laws and regulations and therefore free for general use.

Product liability: The publisher cannot guarantee the accuracy of any information about dosage and application contained in this book. In every individual case the user must check such information by consulting the relevant literature.

Cover design: eStudio Calamar Steinen, Barcelona

Printed on acid-free paper

9 8 7 6 5 4 3 2 1

springer.com

Foreword

Computed tomography has been going through a dramatic evolution of technology in the past years. The increased spatial and temporal resolution directly translate into improved image quality and more versatile applications. Indeed, entirely new areas of clinical application have emerged, one of the most prominent being the recent advent of cardiac computed tomography. Especially CT angiography of the coronary arteries – often referred to as coronary CT angiography – has received tremendous interest and is currently entering the clinical arena. In fact, it has the potential to greatly alter the way in which many patients with suspected coronary artery disease will be worked up. However, the technique is new to the medical community. At this stage, it is crucial that all those potentially involved in the new imaging technology – those who perform and interpret the scan, and also those who order a coronary CT angiogram and advise their patients as to whether a computed tomography examination might be the right test for them – are well informed about the technology and which answers it can provide, about its limitations and problems and about how to best apply it in a given clinical situation.

This is why the textbook edited by Dr. Dewey is most welcome. With ample illustrations, it provides the technological background and principles of scan acquisition and interpretation, as well as examples of clinical applications of coronary CT angiography. May it be a useful resource to its readers and may it contribute towards the further development of this exciting field.

Erlangen, Germany Stephan Achenbach
Baltimore, MD, USA Elliot K. Fishman
April 2008

Acknowledgments

We thank our patients, without whom we would not be able to conduct our clinical work and studies to continuously increase our understanding of the clinical utility of coronary CT angiography.

We are indebted to our technicians and nurses at the Department of Radiology of the Charité – Universitätsmedizin Berlin for their contributions to the success of our clinical cardiovascular imaging program. Without their support, this book would not have been possible. The editorial assistance of Bettina Herwig and Deborah McClellan has been instrumental in writing this book.

The excellent collaboration with the Department of Cardiology and Angiology at the Charité (Chairman: Professor Gert Baumann, Vice Chairman: Professor Karl Stangl) has tremendously facilitated this work. We thank Professor Wolfgang Rutsch, who heads the cardiac catheterization laboratory at the Charité (Campus Mitte), and his coworkers Dr. Adrian Borges, Dr. Hans-Peter Dübel, Dr. Michael Laule, Dr. Christoph Melzer, Professor Verena Stangl, and Professor Heinz Theres for providing the majority of the conventional invasive angiograms presented in this book.

I wholeheartedly thank Drs. Martina and Charles Dewey.

Berlin, Germany Marc Dewey
June 2008

Contents

1 Introduction 1
   B. Hamm

2 Technical and Personnel Requirements 3
   M. Dewey

3 Anatomy 11
   M. Dewey and L.J.M. Kroft

4 CT in the Context of Cardiovascular
   Diagnosis and Management 27
   A.C. Borges and K. Stangl

5 Clinical Indications 31
   M. Dewey

6 Patient Preparation 41
   M. Dewey

7 Examination and Reconstruction 47
   M. Dewey

8a Toshiba Aquilion 64 67
    E. Zimmermann

8b Siemens Somatom Sensation
    and Definition 77
    C. Klessen

8c Philips Brilliance 64 87
    O. Klass and M. Jeltsch

8d General Electric Light Speed VCT 93
    L. Lehmkuhl

9 Reading and Reporting 101
   L.J.M. Kroft and M. Dewey

10 Typical Clinical Examples 129
   M. Dewey

11 Results of Clinical Studies 181
   M. Dewey

12 Outlook 185
   M. Dewey

Index 189

Contributors

Marc Dewey, PD Dr. med.
CharitéCentrum 06 für diagnostische und
interventionelle Radiologie und Nuklearmedizin
Institut für Radiologie
CCM, Charitéplatz 1, 10117 Berlin
Germany
Email: dewey@charite.de

Adrian Constantin Borges, PD Dr. med.
CharitéCentrum 13 für Innere Medizin mit
Kardiologie, Gastroenterologie, Nephrologie
Medizinische Klinik mit Schwerpunkt
Kardiologie und Angiologie
CCM, Charitéplatz 1, 10117 Berlin
Germany
Email: adrian.borges@charite.de

Bernd Hamm, Prof. Dr. med.
CharitéCentrum 06 für diagnostische und
interventionelle Radiologie und Nuklearmedizin
Institut für Radiologie
CCM, Charitéplatz 1, 10117 Berlin
Germany
Email: bernd.hamm@charite.de

Martin Jeltsch, Dr. med.
Klinik für Diagnostische und interventionelle
Radiologie
Universitätsklinikum Ulm
Steinhövelstraße 9, 89075 Ulm
Germany
Email: martin.jeltsch@uniklinik-ulm.de

Oliver Klass, Dr. med.
Klinik für diagnostische und interventionelle Radiologie
Universitätsklinikum Ulm
Steinhövelstraße 9, 89075 Ulm
Germany
Email: oliver.klass@uniklinik-ulm.de

Christian Klessen, Dr. med.
CharitéCentrum 06 für diagnostische und
interventionelle Radiologie und Nuklearmedizin
Institut für Radiologie
CCM, Charitéplatz 1, 10117 Berlin
Germany
Email: christian@klessen.net

Lucia J.M. Kroft, Dr.
Leids Universitair Medisch Centrum
Afdeling Radiologie, Postbus 9600
2300 RC Leiden
The Netherlands
Email: L.J.M.Kroft@lumc.nl

Lukas Lehmkuhl, Dr. med.
Universität Leipzig - Herzzentrum
Diagnostische und Interventionelle Radiologie
Strümpellstrasse 39
04289 Leipzig
Germany
Email: lukas.lehmkuhl@med.uni-leipzig.de

Karl Stangl, Prof. Dr. med.
CharitéCentrum 13 für Innere Medizin mit Kardiologie, Gastroenterologie, Nephrologie
Medizinische Klinik mit Schwerpunkt Kardiologie
und Angiologie
CCM, Charitéplatz 1, 10117 Berlin
Germany
Email: karl.stangl@charite.de

Elke Zimmermann
CharitéCentrum 06 für diagnostische und
interventionelle Radiologie und Nuklearmedizin
Institut für Radiologie
CCM, Charitéplatz 1, 10117 Berlin
Germany
Email: elke.zimmermann@charite.de

Introduction

B. Hamm

The advent of multislice computed tomography was a quantum leap for CT technology. When this technical innovation was first introduced, the radiological community was faced with the task of putting its advantages to use for diagnostic patient management and optimizing its clinical applications. One of the major clinical challenges was to develop this new tool for noninvasive cardiac imaging applications ranging from coronary angiography, to ventricular function analysis, to cardiac valve evaluation.

Marc Dewey and the authors of the book have closely followed the development of this new generation of CT scanners in the clinical setting, in scientific studies and in experimental investigations. The team of authors has gained a wealth of experience spanning CT from 16-slice technology to the most recent generation of 320-slice volume CT scanners. In their scientific investigations, the authors have always placed great emphasis on a critical appraisal of this emerging imaging modality in comparison to well-established diagnostic tests such as coronary angiography, magnetic resonance imaging, and echocardiography, also including the socioeconomic perspective. The close cooperation with the Departments of Cardiology and Cardiac Surgery of the Charité – Universitätsmedizin Berlin was pivotal for obtaining valid results in both clinical examinations and scientific studies and also led to many improvements of the diagnostic workflow.

This book focuses on how to integrate cardiac CT into routine practice. Readers will learn how to perform and interpret coronary CT angiography. A clear overview of the essentials is given, and numerous clinical cardiac CT cases are presented for illustration.

All steps involved in a coronary CT angiography examination are described in detail, including patient preparation, the actual examination, and analysis and interpretation of the findings. Another asset of the book in terms of practical clinical application is that the authors present and discuss the specific features of the CT scanners from all four major vendors as they relate to cardiac imaging. In a final chapter, an outlook is given on conceivable future technical and clinical developments.

I congratulate the team of authors on an excellent book that focuses on the practical clinical aspects of coronary CT angiography and offers its readers an easy to follow introduction to this promising new diagnostic tool. However, the book also provides useful tips and tricks for those already familiar with this imaging modality, which will help them further improve their diagnostic strategy for the benefit of their patients.

Technical and Personnel Requirements

M. Dewey

2.1	Technical Requirements	3
2.2	Purchasing a Scanner	3
2.3	Personnel Requirements	5
2.3.1	Guidelines of the ACR	7
2.3.2	Guidelines of the ACC	8
	Recommended Reading	9

Abstract

In this chapter, we summarize the requirements for setting up a coronary CT angiography practice.

List 2.1. Technical requirements for coronary CT angiography

1. CT scanner with at least 64 simultaneous slices
2. CT scanner with a gantry rotation time of below 400 ms
3. Adaptive multisegment reconstruction or dual-source CT
4. ECG for gating and triggering[a] of acquisitions
5. Dual-head contrast agent injector for saline flush
6. Workstation with automatic curved multiplanar reformation and 3D data segmentation and analysis capabilities

[a] This refers to the acquisition method: retrospective (ECG gating) or prospective (ECG triggering)

2.1 Technical Requirements

Noninvasive coronary angiography is an ascending clinical application that requires very high spatial and temporal resolution. Thus, CT scanners with multiple detector rows (multislice CT [MSCT]), short gantry rotation times, and thin-slice collimation are essential for establishing a successful cardiac CT imaging center. Because 64-slice CT is superior to 16-slice CT in terms of image quality and diagnostic accuracy, we believe that (at least) 64-slice technology is necessary for performing noninvasive coronary angiography (**List 2.1**). CT with 64-slice technology not only increases the quality of the images (**Figs. 2.1–2.3**) but also improves the workflow because scanning and breath-hold times are shorter (**Table 2.1**). The shorter breath-hold time is also very relevant for patients after coronary bypass grafting, for whom 64-slice CT reduces the breath-hold time to about 15 s (**Fig. 2.4**). The faster gantry rotation speed (**List 2.1**) improves temporal resolution and dramatically reduces the likelihood of relevant motion artifacts.

Temporal resolution can be significantly improved by using two simultaneous X-ray sources (dual-source CT, Siemens) and adaptive multisegment reconstruction (Toshiba and Philips). We believe that one of these two approaches should be implemented on cardiac CT scanners to reduce the influence of heart rate on image quality (**List 2.1**). In addition to these technical improvements, beta blocker administration should be used whenever possible to lower the heart rate to below approximately 65 beats per min, because slowing the heart rate to this level further improves both the image quality and the diagnostic accuracy (Chaps. 6 and 7). Finally, an ECG, a dual-head contrast agent injector, and an automatic 3D cardiac analysis workstation are required for cardiac CT (**List 2.1**).

2.2 Purchasing a Scanner

The purchase costs of 16 and 64-slice CT scanners still differ enormously. For applications other than cardiac imaging, 16-slice CT scanners are clearly sufficient to answer the vast majority of clinical questions.

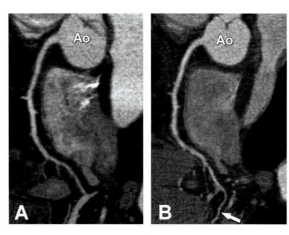

Fig. 2.1 Comparison of 16-slice (**Panel A**) and 64-slice CT coronary angiography (**Panel B**) of the right coronary artery (curved multiplanar reformation) in a 61-year-old male patient. 64-slice CT shows longer vessel segments, especially in the periphery (*arrow*). This enhanced performance can be explained by fewer motion artifacts (due to breathing, extrasystoles, or variations in the length of the cardiac cycle) and the better contrast between arteries and veins resulting from the faster scan and consequently better depiction of the arterial phase. The improved depiction of the arterial phase using 64-slice CT is also demonstrated in **Fig. 2.2**. **Panel B** also illustrates the slightly higher image noise with 64-slice CT, which can be compensated for by the better depiction of the arterial phase and the higher intravascular density. *Ao* aorta

For cardiac applications, however, at least 64-slice technology is clearly needed. The decision to purchase a scanner from any particular manufacturer not only depends on its meeting the relevant technical criteria, such as those mentioned earlier, but will definitely also be influenced by local pricing policies and, more important, by the quality of the maintenance and service support (**List 2.2**). How to perform cardiac CT exams using scanners from different vendors is explained in Chap. 8.

> **List 2.2. Factors to consider in deciding to purchase a particular CT scanner**
>
> 1. Local situation and mixture of different examination types
> 2. Quality of technical and maintenance support
> 3. Availability of high temporal and spatial resolution
> 4. Quality and durability of the application support
> 5. Integration into existing picture archiving and communication systems
> 6. Local pricing policies

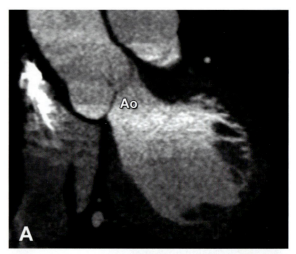

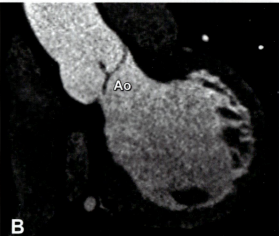

Fig. 2.2 The improved depiction of the arterial phase using 64-slice (**Panel B**), when compared with 16-slice, CT coronary angiography (**Panel A**) is illustrated by a double-oblique coronal slice along the left ventricular outflow tract, with the aortic valve nicely depicted (Ao). In the craniocaudal direction, the density in the aorta and left ventricle shows less variation and decline when 64 simultaneous detector rows are used (**Panel B**). Use of 64-slice CT improves image quality and facilitates the application of automatic coronary vessel and cardiac function analysis tools

Multislice CT has a variety of other applications in addition to cardiac imaging, and CT scanners used solely for cardiac applications are very unlikely to reach the break-even point. Thus, we believe that a mixture of different CT applications is a prerequisite for clinical and economic success. In the US, the Center for Medicare and Medicaid Services (CMS) recently decided after an extensive review that no Medicare national coverage of coronary CT angiography is appropriate at this time. In the decision memo, it is concluded

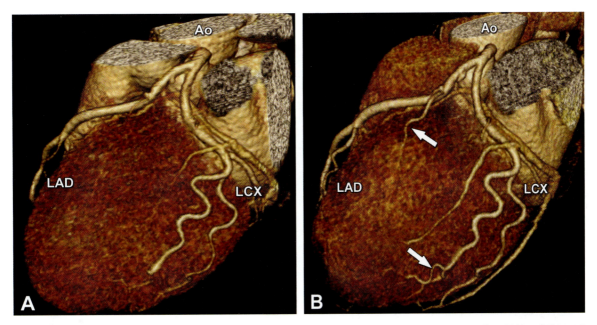

Fig. 2.3 Another example illustrating the improved depiction of distal coronary artery branches using 64-slice CT (**Panel B**) in a 58-year-old female patient. Three-dimensional volume-rendered reconstructions of the left coronary artery with the left anterior descending (LAD) and left circumflex coronary artery (LCX) examined using 16-slice (**Panel A**) and 64-slice CT coronary angiography (**Panel B**). Note the improved depiction of smaller side branches with the 64-slice technology (*arrows* in **Panel B**), when compared with the same segments in 16-slice CT (**Panel A**) *Ao* aorta

that no adequately powered study has established that improved health outcomes can be causally attributed to coronary CT angiography for any well-defined clinical indication. Thus, coverage will be determined by local contractors through the local coverage determination process or case-by-case adjudication. However, the debate is ongoing and further decisions are expected. Chapter 5 presents clinically most relevant indications for coronary CT angiography.

2.3 Personnel Requirements

Having well-trained technicians who are knowledgeable in cardiac CT applications is a prerequisite for success (**List 2.3**). It is better to have a limited number of specialized technicians who perform coronary CT angiography than to have all technicians perform this test. On the one hand, having specialized staff members can ensure a consistently high level of image quality, and these experienced technicians can assist in further educating other coworkers about the entire scanning and reconstruction procedure. On the other hand, if more technicians are involved in performing cardiac CT, coronary CT angiography can easily be offered at night; doing so would, however, also require a physician trained in reading the images. What we consider most helpful in terms of training is to give constant feedback to the technicians about good as well as bad examinations. This approach ensures that a high level of quality is maintained, and small mistakes are prevented from creeping in. Moreover, providing positive feedback about high-quality examinations is very motivating.

> **List 2.3. Personnel requirements for coronary CT angiography**
>
> 1. Well-trained and experienced CT technicians
> 2. Physician knowledgeable in CT and radiation protection
> 3. Physician knowledgeable in cardiac anatomy and pathophysiology
> 4. Team focused on quality assurance

There are two major prerequisites for physicians, in addition to good anatomical, technical (incl. radiation issues), and clinical knowledge: (1) a clear understanding of the entire examination procedure, and (2) the ability

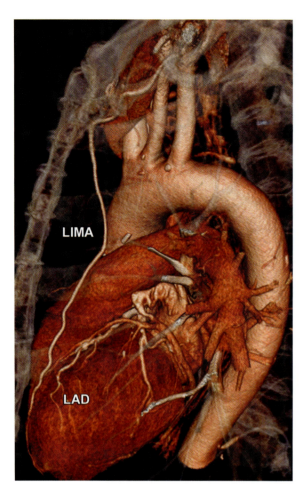

Fig. 2.4 Arterial bypass graft (left internal mammary artery, LIMA), which extends all the way down to the LAD and was scanned in less than 15 s, using a 64-slice CT scanner. With this technology, preoxygenation is no longer necessary for bypass imaging. With 16-slice technology, the scanning took an average of 40–50 s, and preoxygenation was almost always required. Note that CT nicely depicts the distance between the sternum and coronary bypass graft, which can be of relevance if repeat cardiac surgery is considered

Table 2.1 Typical characteristics of 16 and 64-slice CT scanners

	16-slice	64-slice
Slice collimation		
Coronary arteries	0.5–0.75 mm	0.5–0.75 mm
Coronary bypass grafts	0.5–1.25 mm	0.5–0.75 mm
Gantry rotation time		
Coronary angiography	0.4–0.6 s	0.33–0.6 s
Scan length		
Coronary arteries	9–13 cm	Increase by 15%[a]
Coronary bypass grafts	15–22 cm	Increased by 5 to 10%
Effective radiation dose		
Coronary arteries	5–15 mSv	10–20 mSv[b]
Coronary bypass grafts	10–30 mSv	20–40 mSv
Contrast-to-noise ratio		
Coronary angiography	15–25	Similar
Vessel lengths free of motion		
Coronary angiography		Improved by 10–30%[c]
Breath-hold time		
Coronary arteries	25–30 s	8–12 s
Coronary bypass grafts	40–50 s	12–15 s
Contrast agent amount		
Coronary arteries	90–130 ml	60–90 ml
Coronary bypass grafts	130–160 ml	80–110 ml

[a] This increase is due to the larger over-ranging effect of 64-slice CT, which in turn also increases radiation exposure by 15%

[b] The increase in effective dose with 64-slice CT can be explained by the larger over-ranging effect, the fact that scanning cannot be stopped as abruptly once the lower border of the heart has been reached because of the faster table speed, and the higher mA settings necessary (because of the increased scattered radiation and noise with 64-slice CT)

[c] The increase in the visible vessel length free of motion that can be obtained for the three coronary arteries with 64-slice CT scanners is approximately 10% for the left anterior descending, 20% for the left circumflex, and 30% for the right coronary. Most notably, in more than one-third of all cases, the length of the right coronary free of motion is increased by more than 5 cm when 64-slice CT is used

to independently interpret three-dimensional coronary CT angiography datasets on workstations.

Chapters 6 and 7 will discuss how to prepare the patient for coronary CT angiography and how to perform the procedure. Being present during examinations is the key to understanding the work of the technicians and the special requirements of cardiac CT. It is also enlightening for physicians to perform examinations themselves, because doing so can yield important insights into the procedural steps and problems that can be encountered during scanning. This hands-on training also strengthens the position of the physician as an educator of other physicians or technicians. In larger centers, it is good to identify two to three doctors who will be considered the primary contacts for cardiac CT imaging for the technicians as well as the referring physicians.

Competence in image interpretation is best achieved by correlating conventional coronary angiograms with CT angiography results. How to read and interpret cardiac CT scans is explained in Chap. 9. To understand and gain skill in using the workstations, physicians should practice operating them without time pressure. The time necessary to feel comfortable with the workstations will depend on an individual's general computer skills, but 2–4 continuous weeks should be sufficient, and attending one of the true hands-on workshops is a good way to begin the learning process. Such workshops should ideally offer direct comparison of CT findings (on interactive workstations) with conventional angiography findings or the results of cardiac stress tests. This is the only way of acquiring a thorough understanding of coronary and cardiac pathology. Good cardiac CT courses also offer active participation in patient preparation and scanning. Nevertheless, the learning curve for centers with early experience has been shown to last at least 6 months.

However, learning does not stop after a few weeks of intensive familiarization with the workstations or a short course: Even in a team of experienced readers, certain coronary lesions will sometimes be misinterpreted (overcalled or even overlooked). Thus, continuous learning efforts (with comparison of CT to the invasive coronary angiography findings, e.g., in joint interdisciplinary conferences) are necessary to maintain high quality.

There is also a formal accreditation of the physicians' skills and knowledge. The American College of Radiology (ACR) and the American College of Cardiology (ACC) have established guidelines for assessing clinical competence in performing and interpreting cardiac CTs. These guidelines play an increasing role in obtaining certification for coronary CT angiography and claiming reimbursement in the US. Those outside the US may find it useful to study these guidelines as a basis for starting discussions about certification of coronary CT angiography readers and centers in their own countries.

In Germany, for instance, the law requires that every physician performing CT (of any organ) hold the *Fachkunde* ("technical qualification") for CT, which requires having conducted 1,000 examinations over a period of at least 12 months and participating in a course on radiation protection. Such regulations offer promise for increasing radiation safety, and they emphasize the relevance of the ongoing discussion on requirements for coronary CT angiography.

2.3.1 Guidelines of the ACR

Several ACR guidelines are relevant to coronary CT angiography. Most important is the "ACR Practice Guideline for the Performance and Interpretation of

Table 2.2 ACR physician requirements for coronary CT angiography

	Not trained in general or thoracic CT	Board-certified radiologists[a]
CME (category I)	Completion of an ACGME approved training program in the specialty practiced 200 hours in cardiac CT[b]	Training in cardiac CT in an ACGME approved training program 30 h in cardiac anatomy, physiology, pathology, and cardiac CT
Interpretation, reporting, and/or supervised review[c]	500 CT examinations[d]	50 cardiac CT examinations
Maintaining competence	75 contrast-enhanced cardiac CT examinations every 3 years 150 h of CME every 3 years	

ACGME Accreditation Council for Graduate Medical Education

[a] In addition, at least 100 CT examinations are required during each of the past 3 years, as also at least 100 CT examinations per year to maintain competence according to the ACR practice guideline for performing and interpreting diagnostic CT

[b] Including at least 30 h in cardiac anatomy, physiology, pathology, and cardiac CT

[c] Examinations (noncontrast examinations do not count) in a supervised environment during the past 3 years; supervising physician needs to meet the ACR requirements

[d] At least 100 must be a combination of thoracic CT or thoracic CT angiography (exclusive of calcium scoring exams). At least 50 contrast-enhanced cardiac CT examinations must also be included

Cardiac Computed Tomography" (http://www.acr.org/SecondaryMainMenuCategories/quality_safety/guidelines/dx/cardio/ct_cardiac.aspx). Other important guidelines are the "ACR Clinical Statement on Noninvasive Cardiac Imaging," "ACR Practice Guideline for the Performance and Interpretation of CT Angiography," and the "ACR Practice Guideline for Performing and Interpreting Diagnostic Computed Tomography." Later we briefly outline and discuss the recommendations arising from the guidelines that directly relate to coronary CT angiography.

The ACR defines cardiac CT as a chest CT performed primarily for the evaluation of the heart (including the cardiac chambers, valves, myocardium, aorta, central pulmonary vessels, pericardium, coronary arteries, and veins). However, noncardiac structures are included and must be evaluated by a trained physician. Trained physicians are defined in the "ACR Practice Guideline for Performing and Interpreting Diagnostic Computed Tomography" as board-certified radiologists who have interpreted and reported at least 100 CT examinations over each of the past 3 years and interpret and report at least 100 CT examinations per year to maintain competence. These physicians can achieve competence in the performance and interpretation of coronary CT angiography by at least 30 h of CME in cardiac anatomy, physiology, pathology, and cardiac CT, plus the interpretation, reporting, and/or supervised review of at least 50 cardiac CT examinations during the past 3 years (**Table 2.2**). Physicians who are not defined in this guideline as trained physicians in diagnostic CT can achieve competence in the performance and interpretation of coronary CT angiography by at least 200 h of CME in the performance and interpretation of cardiac CT, plus the interpretation, reporting, and/or supervised review of at least 500 chest CT examinations (including 50 cardiac CT examinations) during the past 3 years (**Table 2.2**). The ACR stresses that all physicians performing cardiac CT need to be knowledgeable about the administration, risks, and contraindications of beta blockers and nitroglycerin.

2.3.2 Guidelines of the ACC

The "ACC Clinical Competence Statement on Cardiac Imaging with Computed Tomography and Magnetic Resonance" (http://www.acc.org/qualityandscience/clinical/competence/imaging/index.pdf) states that it is intended to be complementary to the recommendations of the ACR on noninvasive cardiac imaging. Cardiac CT is defined in this guideline as the imaging of anatomy, function, coronary calcium, noncalcified plaque, and congenital heart disease. The guideline defines three levels of competence in coronary CT angiography, of which two are relevant here. Level 2 allows independent performance and interpretation of cardiac CT and requires 8 weeks (each consisting of at least 35 h) of cumulative training in a clinical cardiac CT laboratory plus 150 contrast-enhanced and 50

Table 2.3 ACC physician requirements for coronary CT angiography

	Level 2[a]	Level 3[b]
CME (category I)	20 h in cardiac CT	40 h in cardiac CT
Training[c]	8 weeks	6 months
Interpretation, reporting, and/or supervised review	50 noncontrast cardiac CT examinations 150 contrast-enhanced cardiac CT examinations[d]	100 noncontrast cardiac CT examinations 300 contrast-enhanced cardiac CT examinations[d]
Maintaining competence	50 contrast-enhanced cardiac CT examinations every year 20 h of CME in cardiac CT every 3 years	100 contrast-enhanced cardiac CT examinations every year 40 h of CME in cardiac CT every 3 years

[a] Allows independent performance and interpretation of cardiac CT

[b] Allows serving as a director of an independent cardiac CT center

[c] Training must be conducted under the supervision of a level 3 physician. Each week consists of at least 35 h. The time commitment does not go into effect until July 2010

[d] Physically present and involved in the acquisition, performance, and interpretation of 50 (level 2) or 100 (level 3) contrast-enhanced cardiac CT examinations. The noncontrast examinations can be performed in the same patients who undergo contrast-enhanced CT

noncontrast cardiac CT examinations. A physician willing to achieve level 2 competence needs to be physically present and involved in the acquisition and performance of 50 of the 150 contrast-enhanced cardiac CT examinations (**Table 2.3**). Level 3 allows serving as a director of an independent cardiac CT center and requires 6 months of cumulative training in a clinical cardiac CT laboratory plus 300 contrast-enhanced and 100 noncontrast cardiac CT examinations. A physician willing to achieve level 3 competence needs to be physically present and involved in the acquisition and performance of 100 of the 300 contrast-enhanced cardiac CT examinations (**Table 2.3**). An additional recommendation for "Training in Advanced Cardiovascular Imaging (Computed Tomography)" has been released by the ACC. The ACC stresses that all physicians performing cardiac CT need to be knowledgeable about radiation risks and noncardiac findings on coronary CT angiography.

Recommended Reading

1. Budoff MJ, Achenbach S, Berman DS, et al. Task force 13: training in advanced cardiovascular imaging (computed tomography) endorsed by the American Society of Nuclear Cardiology, Society of Atherosclerosis Imaging and Prevention, Society for Cardiovascular Angiography and Interventions, and Society of Cardiovascular Computed Tomography. J Am Coll Cardiol 2008; 51:409–14
2. Budoff MJ, Cohen MC, Garcia MJ, et al. ACCF/AHA clinical competence statement on cardiac imaging with computed tomography and magnetic resonance. J Am Coll Cardiol 2005; 46:383–402
3. Chin S, Ong T, Chan W, et al. 64 row multi-detector computed tomography coronary image from a centre with early experience: first illustration of learning curve. J Geriatric Cardiology 2006; 3:29–34
4. Dewey M, Hamm B. Cost effectiveness of coronary angiography and calcium scoring using CT and stress MRI for diagnosis of coronary artery disease. Eur Radiol 2007; 17:1301–9
5. Dewey M, Hoffmann H, Hamm B. CT coronary angiography using 16 and 64 simultaneous detector rows: intraindividual comparison. Fortschr Röntgenstr 2007; 179:581–86
6. Hamon M, Morello R, Riddell JW. Coronary arteries: diagnostic performance of 16 versus 64-section spiral CT compared with invasive coronary angiography–meta-analysis. Radiology 2007; 245:720–31
7. Hausleiter J, Meyer T, Hadamitzky M, et al. Non-invasive coronary computed tomographic angiography for patients with suspected coronary artery disease: the Coronary Angiography by Computed Tomography with the Use of a Submillimeter resolution (CACTUS) trial. Eur Heart J 2007; 28:3034–41
8. Jacobs JE, Boxt LM, Desjardins B, Fishman EK, Larson PA, Schoepf J. ACR practice guideline for the performance and interpretation of cardiac computed tomography (CT). J Am Coll Radiol 2006; 3:677–85
9. Pannu HK, Alvarez W, Jr., Fishman EK. Beta-blockers for cardiac CT: a primer for the radiologist. AJR Am J Roentgenol 2006; 186: S341–5
10. Weinreb JC, Larson PA, Woodard PK, et al. ACR clinical statement on noninvasive cardiac imaging. J Am Coll Radiol 2005; 2:471–7

The ACR practice guideline for the performance and interpretation of cardiac CT (Jacobs et al.) can be accessed at:
http://www.acr.org/SecondaryMainMenuCategories/quality_safety/guidelines/dx/cardio/ct_cardiac.aspx
The guideline of the ACC (Budoff et al.) can be accessed at:
http://www.acc.org/qualityandscience/clinical/competence/imaging/index.pdf
http://www.escr.org
http://www.nasci.org
http://www.scct.org

Anatomy

M. Dewey and L.J.M. Kroft

3.1 Coronary Arteries 11
3.1.1 Coronary Artery Dominance 13
3.1.2 Coronary Artery Segments 17
3.1.3 Frequent Coronary Artery Variants 22
3.2 Myocardium 25
Recommended Reading 26

Abstract

This chapter reviews coronary and myocardial anatomy and stresses its relevance to CT cardiac imaging.

3.1 Coronary Arteries

The major coronary arteries, together with their second-order branches, can usually be well-visualized by MSCT. Third-order branches may be visualized, but smaller branches are generally not visible because of their small size and the limitations of the scanner with regard to spatial and temporal resolution.

In the normal situation, the coronary arteries arise from the proximal aorta. The right and left coronary arteries arise from the right and left sinus of Valsalva, respectively. The noncoronary sinus of Valsalva is usually the posterior one. The main coronary artery segments run in the left and right atrioventricular grooves between the atria and ventricles, and then perpendicularly in the anterior and posterior interventricular grooves between the left and right ventricles (**Fig. 3.1**). The coronary arteries and their side branches vary greatly in terms of their presence or absence and their size, shape, and length.

The right coronary artery (RCA) arises from the aorta at the right sinus of Valsalva and courses in the right atrioventricular groove. Along its course, it first gives off the conus artery (in 50% of all individuals; in the other 50%, the conus artery arises directly from the aorta). It then gives off the sinoatrial node artery (in roughly 60%; in the remaining individuals, it arises from the left circumflex coronary artery [LCX]). Acute marginal branches arise from the mid-segment and posterior right ventricular branches from the distal segment. In case of a right-dominant circulation, the RCA gives rise to the posterior descending artery at or near the crux cordis (where the left and right atrioventricular groove and posterior interventricular groove join). The posterior descending artery courses in the posterior interventricular groove, and the RCA gives rise to posterolateral artery branches as it continues in the left atrioventicular groove beyond the crux. The RCA supplies both the myocardium of the right atrium and ventricle and posterior portions of the left ventricle and interventricular septum.

The left main coronary artery (LM) arises from the aorta at the left sinus of Valsalva and has a length that varies from 0–15 mm. The LM usually bifurcates into the left anterior descending coronary artery (LAD) and LCX; however, in a third of the population, the LM ends as a trifurcation with an intermediate branch (IMB, also called ramus medianus) arising between the LAD and the LCX (**Fig. 3.2**). An IMB can be regarded as a diagonal branch or as an obtuse marginal branch, depending on its course along the left ventricle. In about 1% of the population, the LM is absent, and there are separate ostia for the LAD and LCX (**Fig. 3.2**).

The LAD courses in the anterior interventricular groove. The major branches of the LAD are the septal branches that pass downward into the interventricular septum and the diagonal branches (usually one to three

12 Chapter 3 • Anatomy

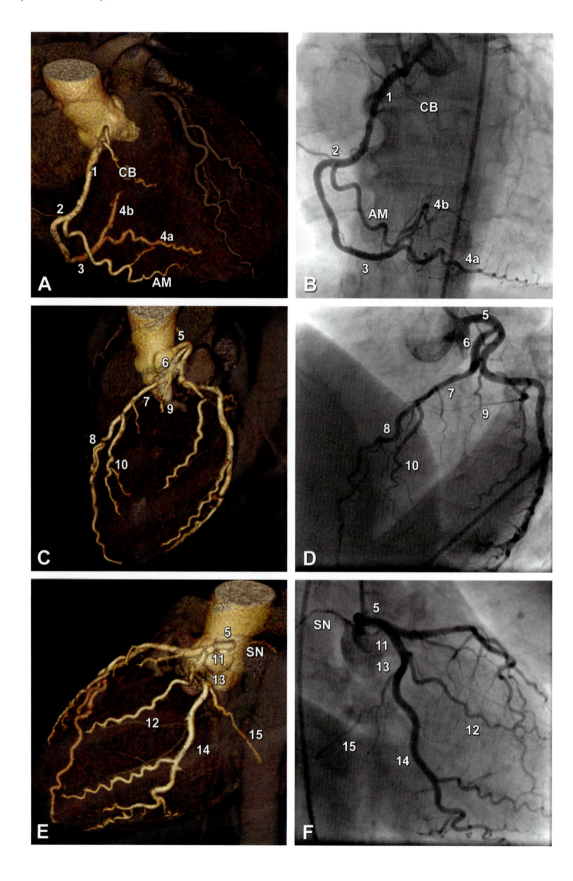

3.1 • Coronary Arteries

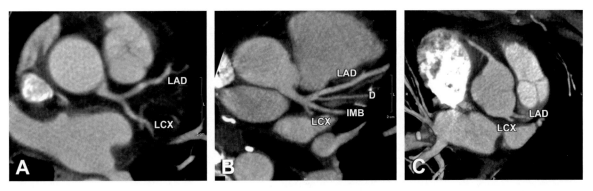

Fig. 3.2 Different types of left main coronary artery bifurcation. Oblique transverse thin-slab maximum-intensity projection images. The left main coronary artery is shown bifurcating into the left anterior descending coronary artery (LAD) and LCX (**Panel A**), the left main with trifurcation into the LAD and the LCX, and in between an intermediate branch (IMB, **Panel B**). Note the high diagonal branch (D) from the LAD (**Panel B**). An absent left main coronary artery, with separate origins for the LAD and LCX (**Panel C**)

are present) that pass over the anterolateral aspect of the heart. The LAD and its side branches supply the anterior as well as the anteroseptal and anterolateral left ventricular segments. The septal branches, in particular, serve as important collateral pathways.

The LCX courses in the left atrioventricular groove, where the major side branches are the obtuse marginal branches (usually one to three are present) that supply the lateral free wall of the left ventricle. The left atrial circumflex branches that supply the lateral and posterior aspect of the left atrium also arise from the LCX.

3.1.1 Coronary Artery Dominance

The circulation is right-dominant in about 60–85% of the population (the RCA gives rise to the posterior descending and at least one posterolateral branch). Left coronary dominance (the LCX gives rise to the posterior descending branch) is found in 7–20% of the population, whereas a balanced (or codominant) distribution is seen in 7–20% (the RCA gives rise to the posterior descending, and the LCX gives rise to posterolateral branches). In the case of a left-dominant circulation, the RCA is small and does not supply blood to the left ventricular myocardium. Recognizing the dominancy of the circulation is important, so as to avoid confusing this situation with branch occlusion (e.g., a short RCA in a left-dominant circulation, **Fig. 3.3**). Although it is the RCA that is typically dominant, it is usually the left coronary artery that supplies the major part of the left ventricular myocardium as well as the anterior and mid portions of the interventricular septum.

Fig. 3.1 Direct comparison of segmental coronary artery anatomy, as depicted by multislice CT (*left panels*, three-dimensional reconstructions) and conventional coronary angiography (*right panels*). The RCA is shown in **Panels A** and **B**, and the left coronary artery with its two main branches – the left anterior descending and the left circumflex – in **Panels C–F**. The RCA (**Panels A** and **B**) is composed of segments 1–4, with the distal segment (4) being further subdivided into 4a (posterior descending artery) and 4b (right posterolateral branch). The left main coronary artery (**Panels C–F**) is referred to as segment 5, and the left anterior descending coronary artery (**Panels C** and **D**) is composed of segments 6–10, with the two diagonal branches being segments 9 and 10. The LCX (**Panels E** and **F**) is composed of segments 11–15, with the two (obtuse) marginal branches being segments 12 and 14. Note that the distal left circumflex (segment 15) is rather small in this patient with a right-dominant coronary circulation. The sinus node artery (SN) is the first branch of the LCX in this patient (**Panels E** and **F**) but is more commonly one of the first branches of the RCA. *AM* acute marginal branch; *CB* conus branch. **Table 3.1** gives an overview of all coronary artery segment numbers and names

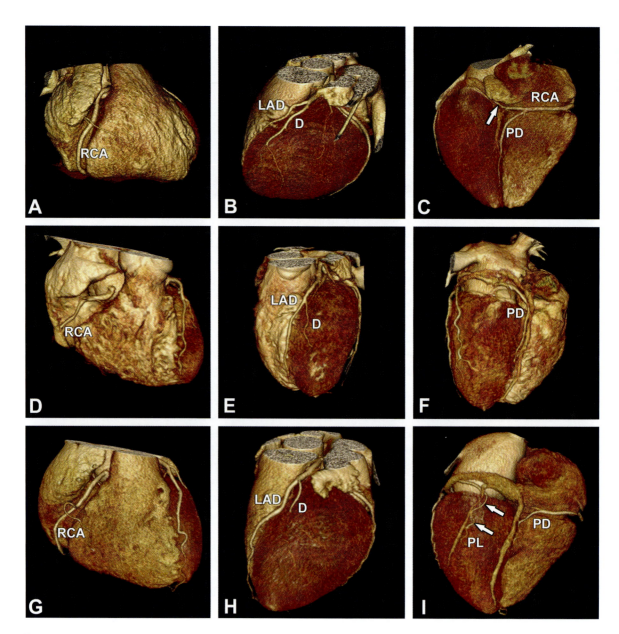

Fig. 3.3 Different coronary artery distribution types on three-dimensional volume-rendered images. **Panels A–C**: Right-dominant circulation. The RCA is dominant and gives rise to the posterior descending artery (PD), and also continues in the left atrioventricular groove (*arrow* in **Panel C**). **Panels D–F**: Left-dominant circulation. The LCX is dominant and gives rise to the posterior descending artery (PD in **Panel F**). Note the small RCA in the left-dominant coronary artery system (**Panel D**). **Panels G–I**: Balanced circulation (codominant circulation), where the RCA gives rise to the PD and the LCX gives rise to a posterolateral branch (PL in **Panel I**). *D* diagonal branch; *LAD* left anterior descending artery

3.1 • Coronary Arteries

Table 3.1 Coronary artery segmental anatomy[a]

Segment no.	Vessel name	Segment name
1	Right coronary artery (RCA)	Proximal right coronary
2		Mid right coronary
3		Distal right coronary
4a		Posterior descending artery[b]
4b		Right posterolateral branch[b]
5	Left main coronary artery (LM)	Left main coronary artery
6	Left anterior descending artery (LAD)	Proximal left anterior descending
7		Mid left anterior descending
8		Distal left anterior descending
9		First diagonal branch
10		Second diagonal branch
11	Left circumflex artery (LCX)	Proximal left circumflex
12		First (obtuse) marginal
13		Mid left circumflex
14		Second (obtuse) marginal
15		Distal left circumflex[b]
16	Ramus intermedius[c]	Ramus intermedius[c]

[a] This segmentation is based on the AHA segmentation published in 1975 by Austen et al.

[b] In case of RCA dominance, at least one right posterolateral branch (segment 4b) is present and supplies the inferolateral myocardial segments. If the left coronary artery is dominant, the distal LCX ends as the posterior descending coronary artery (segment 4a). In case of codominance, segment 4a is part of the RCA, and the distal left circumflex ends as a posterolateral branch after giving off two marginal branches

[c] A ramus intermedius (intermediate) branch is present in approximately 30% of patients

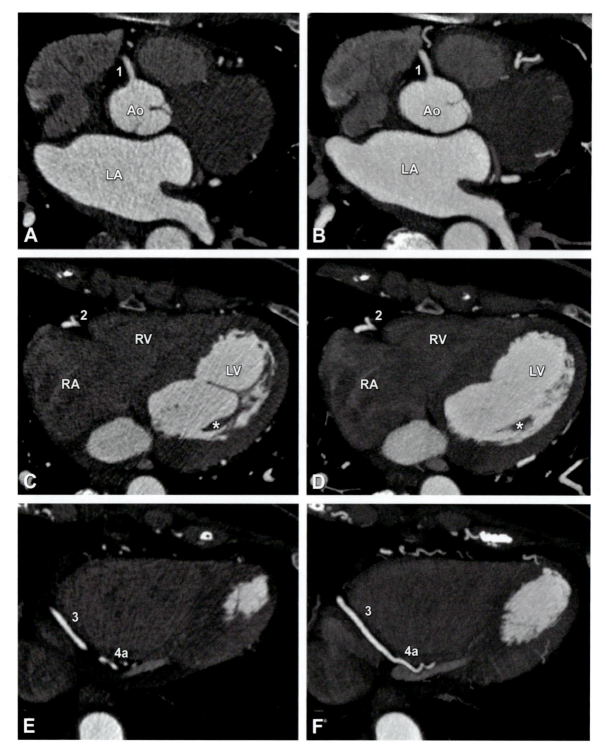

Fig. 3.4 Caption see opposite page

3.1 · Coronary Arteries

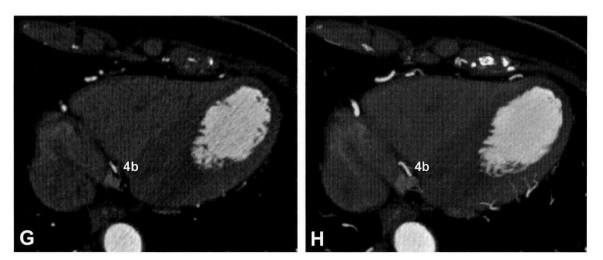

Fig. 3.4 The RCA with all its segments in axial slices (*left panels*), and the corresponding maximum-intensity projections of 5-mm thickness in the axial orientation for comparison (*right panels*). The proximal segment of the RCA (1) comes off the aorta, arising from the right sinus of Valsalva (**Panels A** and **B**). It first moves anteriorly and then (as segment 2) caudally in the right atrioventricular sulcus (**Panels C** and **D**) to the posterior surface of the heart (**Panels E** and **F**), where it again moves in the horizontal plane on the diaphragmatic face of the heart as segment 3. At the crux cordis, segment 3 bifurcates into the posterior descending artery (4a) and the right posterolateral branch (4b in **Panels G** and **H**). In cases of dominance of the RCA (as in this case), segments 4a and b are side branches of the RCA. In case of left coronary artery dominance, the posterior descending artery (4a) is part of the LCX. *Ao* aorta; *LA* left atrium; *LV* left ventricle; *RA* right atrium; *RV* right ventricle

3.1.2 Coronary Artery Segments

The coronary arteries with their side branches can be further subdivided and classified (**Figs. 3.1, 3.4–3.6** and **Table 3.1**). These segments are of tremendous importance in describing the location of significant coronary stenoses found on noninvasive imaging and correlating them with possible myocardial ischemia, as well as for accurately guiding subsequent revascularization. Use of the 17-segment model further described in **Table 3.1** and **Figs. 3.1, 3.4–3.6** is recommended for this purpose; in the case of pathology (i.e., the presence of stenoses), it is recommended that the location be reported by segment name or number. The 17-segment model has several advantages over its competitor segmentation schemes, the foremost of which are its simplicity and conciseness.

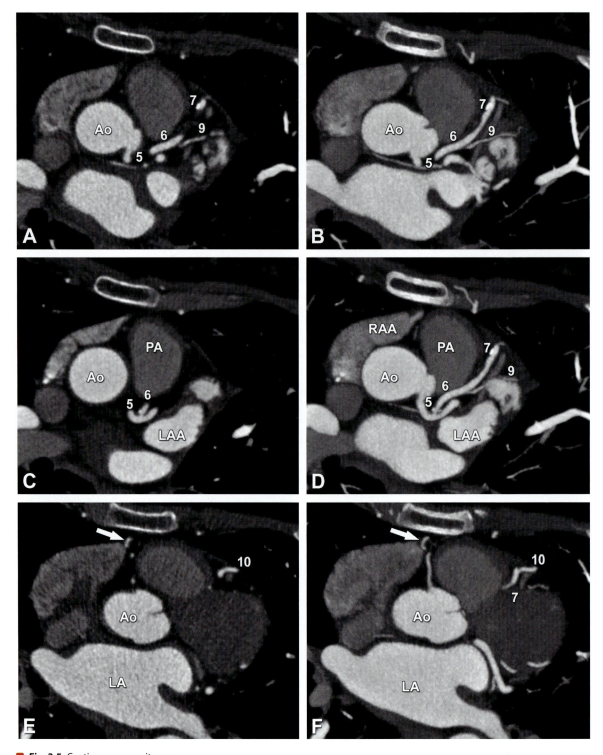

Fig. 3.5 Caption see opposite page

3.1 · Coronary Arteries

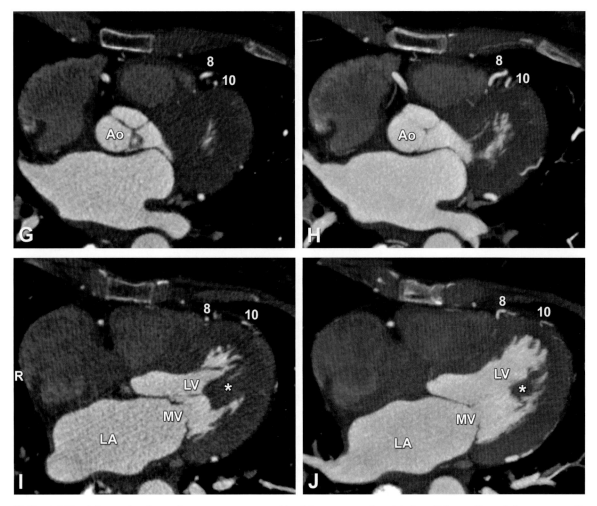

Fig. 3.5 The left anterior descending coronary artery with all its segments in axial slices (*left panels*), and the corresponding maximum-intensity projections of 5-mm thickness in the axial orientation for comparison (*right panels*). The proximal left anterior descending coronary artery segment (6) is the anterior branch of the left main coronary artery (5, **Panels A–D**). Segment 6 of the left anterior descending coronary artery then bifurcates into the mid-left anterior descending (7) and the first diagonal branch (9, **Panels A–D**). Further caudally, the mid-left anterior descending coronary artery gives off the distal segment (8) and the second diagonal (10, **Panels E–J**) In **Panels E** and **F**, the conus branch (*arrows*, first side branch of the RCA), which travels cranial to the proximal RCA segment, is also visible. *Ao* aorta; *Asterisk* papillary muscles; *LAA* left atrial appendage; *LA* left atrium; *LV* left ventricle; *MV* mitral valve; *PA* pulmonary artery; *RAA* right atrial appendage

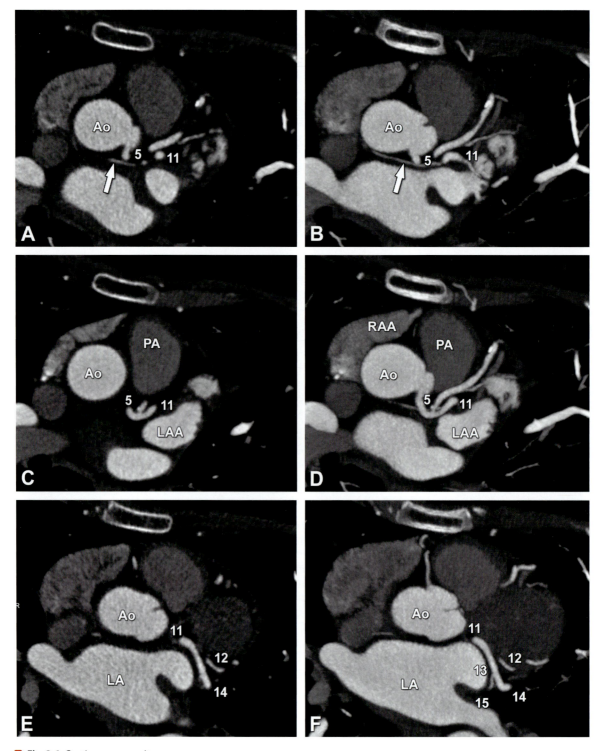

◘ **Fig. 3.6** Caption see opposite page

3.1 · Coronary Arteries

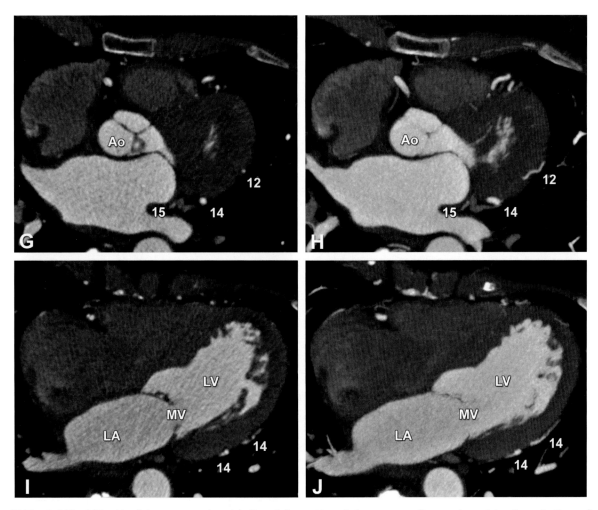

Fig. 3.6 The LCX with all its segments in axial slices (*left panels*), and the corresponding maximum-intensity projections of 5-mm thickness in the axial orientation for comparison (*right panels*). The proximal LCX segment (11) is the posterior branch of the left main coronary artery (5, **Panels A–D**). Further down, the proximal left circumflex splits into the mid-left circumflex (13) and the first (obtuse) marginal branch (12, **Panels E–H**). The mid-left circumflex (13) then gives off the distal left circumflex (15, **Panels F–H**) (obtuse) marginal branches (14, **Panels E–J**), which supply the inferolateral myocardial segments In the case of left coronary artery dominance, the distal circumflex (15) ends as the posterior descending artery (4a), whereas in right coronary dominance, as in this case, the RCA gives rise to the posterior descending and at least one posterolateral branch. The sinus node artery (*arrow* in **Panels A** and **B**) is the first branch of the LCX in this patient. *Ao* aorta; *Asterisk* papillary muscles; *LAA* left atrial appendage; *LA* left atrium; *LV* left ventricle; *MV* mitral valve; *PA* pulmonary artery; *RAA* right atrial appendage

3.1.3 Frequent Coronary Artery Variants

In addition to the variation in normal anatomy caused by left or right dominance, there are other variations, such as myocardial bridging and anomalous origin, as well as variability in the course of the coronary arteries.

In less than 5% of patients, interventional coronary angiography identifies myocardial bridging. This term refers to the descent of a portion of the coronary artery into the myocardium (**Fig. 3.7**). Because of the improved imaging of myocardial tissue that can be achieved with MSCT coronary angiography, myocardial bridging can be observed in about 30% of patients when this technique is used, a figure that is consistent with most pathological reports. Myocardial bridging is usually confined to the LAD, diagonal or IM branches. At systole, the overlying bridge of myocardial tissue contracts and may cause systolic compression of the coronary artery segment. At diastole, the caliber is generally normal. Because most of the flow through the coronary arteries occurs at diastole, myocardial bridging does not usually cause symptoms. However, incidental cases have been associated with ischemia.

The anomalous origin or course of a coronary artery is less frequently encountered (<1%). The existence of separate origins for the LAD and LCX has already been discussed. The two most frequent other anomalies are an RCA with an anomalous origin from the LM or the left sinus of Valsalva, and an LCX with an anomalous origin from the RCA or the right sinus of Valsalva.

In the case of an anomalous origin of the RCA from the left sinus of Valsalva or LM, the RCA commonly courses anteriorly between the aorta and the pulmonary trunk (**Fig. 3.8**). This inter-arterial course is also called "malignant course," because these patients have a high risk for exercise-induced ischemia and sudden death. At exercise, more blood is present in the aorta and pulmonary artery, causing the anomalous segment to be squeezed between these large arteries and potentially inducing ischemia. Also, the anomalous artery is usually somewhat narrowed at the origin and forms an acute angle with the aorta that may be pinched off by exercise. Other (left coronary artery) anomalies with an inter-arterial course between the aorta and pulmonary trunk can also cause ischemia.

The most frequent LCX anomaly is an LCX having its origin from the RCA or right sinus of Valsalva, where the LCX courses posterior to the aorta to enter its normal location in the left atrioventricular groove (**Fig. 3.9**). This is a benign condition that is not associated with ischemia.

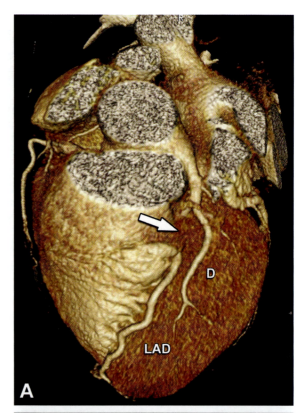

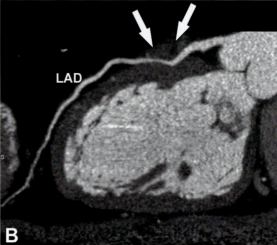

Fig. 3.7 Myocardial bridging of a proximal left anterior descending coronary artery (LAD) segment (*arrows*). Three-dimensional volume-rendered image (**Panel A**) and curved multiplanar reformation (**Panel B**). Note the bridge of myocardial tissue overlying the LAD segment (*arrows*, **Panel B**). *D* diagonal branch

3.1 · Coronary Arteries

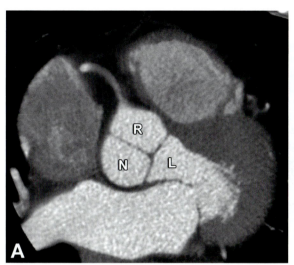
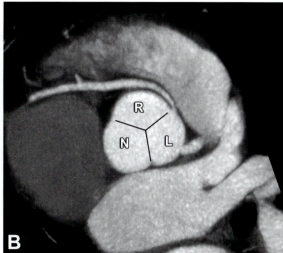

Fig. 3.8 Normal origin of the RCA, arising from the right sinus of Valsalva (**Panel A**), in an oblique transverse thin-slab maximum-intensity projection image. Anomalous origin of the RCA, arising from the left sinus of Valsalva, with an inter-arterial course between the aorta and pulmonary trunk (**Panel B**). *L* left sinus of Valsalva; *R* right sinus of Valsalva; *N* non-coronary sinus

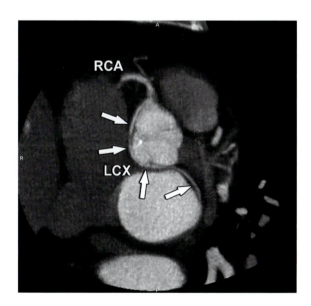

Fig. 3.9 LCX with an anomalous origin, arising at the origin of the RCA, as shown in an oblique transverse thin-slab maximum-intensity projection image. The LCX follows a retro-aortic course to its normal position in the left atrioventricular groove (*arrows*). This is a benign variant that is not associated with ischemia

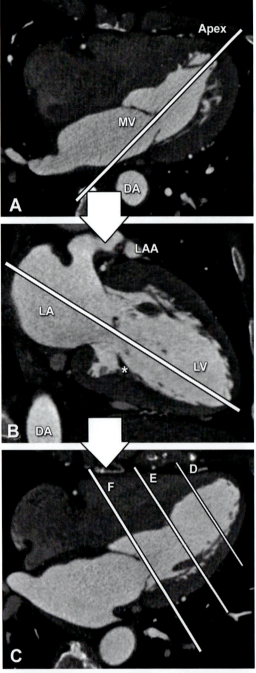

Fig. 3.10 Generating short and long-axis views for cardiac function analysis. On the basis of an axial CT slice (**Panel A**), a two-chamber view (**Panel B**) along the left ventricle (LV) and left atrium (LA) is created by connecting the apex of the left ventricle with the mitral valve (MV; white line in **Panel A**). From this two-chamber view, a four-chamber view is generated (**Panel C**) by again connecting the apex of the left ventricle with the mitral valve (MV). In this way, the individual double-oblique cardiac long axes can be identified. True cardiac short-axis slices are created by further reformations orthogonal to the interventricular septum (**Panels D–F**). In this way, apical (**Panel D**), mid-cavity (**Panel E**), and basal (**Panel F**) short-axis slices are created, for instance, to assess global and regional cardiac function; they can be viewed as cine loops throughout the cardiac cycle. *Asterisk* papillary muscles; *DA* descending aorta; *LAA* left atrial appendage; *LA* left atrium; *LV* left ventricle

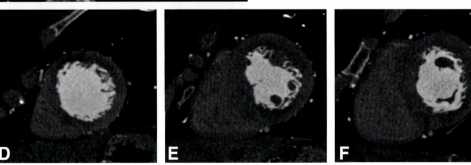

3.2 Myocardium

In addition to the coronary artery anatomy described in the previous section, a basic understanding of gross cardiac anatomy is necessary for reporting cardiac function analysis using multislice CT. **Figure 3.10** describes how short and long axes orthogonal to the cardiac structures can be reconstructed from axial CT data sets. We recommend using the 17-segment model for reporting myocardial findings (**Fig. 3.11**), and for practical purposes it seems more convenient to use the myocardial segment names instead of the segment numbers (**Table 3.2**).

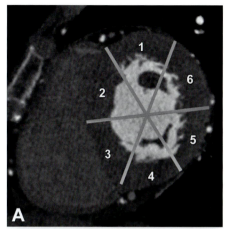
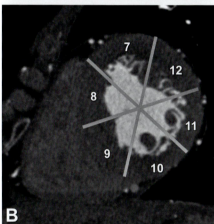
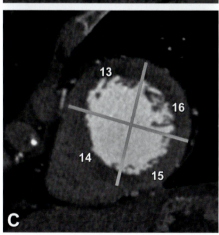

Fig. 3.11 Segmental myocardial anatomy, as shown in true cardiac short-axis slices. The basal short axis is divided into segments 1–6, in counter-clockwise order (**Panel A**). The mid-cavity (**Panel B**) and apical segments (**Panel C**) are also numbered in counter-clockwise order with the numbers 7–12 and 13–17, respectively. Segment 17 is not displayed in the apical short-axis slice because it represents the apex, which is nicely seen in the long-axis views in **Panels B** and **C** of **Fig. 3.10**. The myocardial segment names and numbers are given in **Table 3.2**

Table 3.2 Myocardial segmental anatomy[a]

Segment no.	Location	Segment name
1	Basal	Anterior
2		Anteroseptal
3		Inferoseptal
4		Inferior
5		Inferolateral
6		Anterolateral
7	Mid-Cavity	Anterior
8		Anteroseptal
9		Inferoseptal
10		Inferior
11		Inferolateral
12		Anterolateral
13	Apical	Anterior
14		Septal
15		Inferior
16		Lateral
17	Apical	Apex

[a] AHA segmentation published in 2002 by Cerqueira et al.

Recommended Reading

1. Austen WG, Edwards JE, Frye RL, et al. A reporting system on patients evaluated for coronary artery disease. Report of the Ad Hoc Committee for Grading of Coronary Artery Disease, Council on Cardiovascular Surgery, American Heart Association. Circulation 1975; 51:5–40
2. Boxt LM. CT. Anatomy of the heart. Int J Cardiovasc Imaging 2005; 21:13–27
3. Cerqueira MD, Weissman NJ, Dilsizian V, et al. Standardized myocardial segmentation and nomenclature for tomographic imaging of the heart: a statement for healthcare professionals from the Cardiac Imaging Committee of the Council on Clinical Cardiology of the American Heart Association. Circulation 2002; 105:539–42
4. Kini S, Bis KG, Weaver L. Normal and variant coronary arterial and venous anatomy on high-resolution CT angiography. AJR Am J Roentgenol 2007; 188:1665–74
5. Konen E, Goitein O, Sternik L, Eshet Y, Shemesh J, Di Segni E. The prevalence and anatomical patterns of intramuscular coronary arteries: a coronary computed tomography angiographic study. J Am Coll Cardiol 2007; 49:587–93
6. Krakau I, Lapp H. Das Herzkatheterbuch. Stuttgart: Thieme, 2005
7. Levin DC, Harrington DP, Bettmann MA, Garnic JD, Davidoff A, Lois J. Anatomic variations of the coronary arteries supplying the anterolateral aspect of the left ventricle: possible explanation for the "Unexplained" anterior aneurysm. Invest Radiol 1982; 17:458–62
8. O'Brien JP, Srichai MB, Hecht EM, Kim DC, Jacobs JE. Anatomy of the heart at multidetector CT: what the radiologist needs to know. Radiographics 2007; 27:1569–82
9. Popma J. Coronary angiography and intravascular ultrasound imaging. In: Zipes DP, ed. Braunwald's heart disease: a textbook of cardiovascular medicine. Philadelphia: Elsevier; 2005
10. Saremi F, Abolhoda A, Ashikyan O, et al. Arterial supply to sinuatrial and atrioventricular nodes: imaging with multidetector CT. Radiology 2008; 246:99–107; discussion 08–9
11. Schmitt R, Froehner S, Brunn J, et al. Congenital anomalies of the coronary arteries: imaging with contrast-enhanced, multidetector computed tomography. Eur Radiol 2005; 15:1110–21
12. Yamanaka O, Hobbs RE. Coronary artery anomalies in 126,595 patients undergoing coronary arteriography. Cathet Cardiovasc Diagn 1990; 21:28–40
13. Zimmermann E, Schnapauff D, Dewey M. Cardiac and coronary anatomy in CT. Semin Ultrasound CT MR 2008; 29:176–81

CT in the Context of Cardiovascular Diagnosis and Management

A.C. Borges and K. Stangl

4.1 CT as a Supplement to Other Noninvasive Imaging Tests 27
4.2 Role of CT in Clinical Cardiology 27
4.3 CT as a Screening Test: Indications in Asymptomatic Individuals? 28
4.4 Risk-Benefit of Cardiac CT: Economic and Biological Costs of Cardiac Imaging............ 29
    Recommended Reading............................... 29

Abstract

CT coronary imaging has emerged as a reliable diagnostic method for detecting significant coronary stenoses in selected patients.

4.1 CT as a Supplement to Other Noninvasive Imaging Tests

Echocardiography is the most important and the first-line noninvasive imaging method in cardiology and intensive care medicine, supplemented in special clinical situations by magnetic resonance imaging (MRI). There are a number of reasons for the first-line use of echocardiography: It offers a noninvasive approach, without radiation exposure; it does not involve renal clearance of the contrast medium; it is available in intensive care units, emergency and operating rooms; and extensive education and training in this technique is offered in most European and American countries.

However, despite these advantages, echocardiography and MRI have recognized weaknesses in terms of calcium detection, plaque characterization, imaging of the pulmonary circulation, and direct visualization of the coronary arteries or bypass grafts and collaterals. Multislice CT is more sensitive than MRI and is equally specific in the detection of significant (>50% diameter) stenoses of the coronary arteries. However, if many patients need invasive coronary angiography after positive CT coronary angiography, the additional contrast and radiation exposure incurred strongly argues against using CT angiography.

4.2 Role of CT in Clinical Cardiology

Assessing the clinical significance of stenotic lesions requires the integration of cardiac anatomy with the functional consequences of that anatomy. Functional imaging is performed using nuclear cardiology (myocardial scintigraphy), stress echocardiography, and cardiovascular MRI. These imaging techniques detect stress-induced wall motion or perfusion abnormalities as markers of ischemia and have high diagnostic accuracy for detecting coronary artery disease (CAD). A normal study does not exclude coronary artery stenoses, but rather excludes lesions resulting in ischemia.

A variety of CT techniques are available for the evaluation of CAD. In addition to coronary calcium scoring, CT allows direct evaluation of the coronary arteries and the severity of stenosis. This diagnostic capability has attracted considerable attention because these CT techniques allow angiography to be performed noninvasively. Metaanalyses have demonstrated excellent diagnostic accuracy, with a mean per-patient sensitivity of 97% and specificity of 78% (Chap. 11). The high sensitivity reflects a high accuracy in excluding CAD, and recent studies have shown high negative predictive values of 95% on a per-patient basis. The introduction of 16-slice and 64-slice scanners has resulted in an increased accuracy in both the detection and exclusion of CAD. Although the high diagnostic accuracy of CT is well established, the most important question, clinically speaking, is: Which patients should undergo noninvasive coronary angiography with CT?

Much of the existing research is limited by preselection bias. Most of the studies thus far have been performed in patients with a high pretest likelihood of CAD. In the future, CT may serve as a *gatekeeper* or *filter* for invasive angiography: The higher accuracy of 16-slice and 64-slice scanners will virtually exclude false-negative CT studies. Thus, CT before valve surgery, for example, may be useful in ruling out significant artery stenoses, with an acceptable negative predictive value. Although CT seems to have limited value in most candidates for invasive coronary angiography, there is another important subset of patients to be considered: those with atypical angina pectoris. As previously demonstrated, negative results on CT angiography are associated with a posttest probability of CAD that is below 10% in patients with pretest probabilities of less than 70%. Only in patients with a pretest probability below 30% (i.e., in patients with unspecific chest pain and negative or equivocal results on noninvasive stress tests) does CT achieve a posttest probability below 5% after a negative test. However, appropriate use of CT in such patients requires a careful clinical workup with functional tests because of the potentially rather low positive predictive value of CT.

In addition to coronary angiography and plaque composition assessment, other applications of CT that may be relevant are the evaluation of valvular and pericardial calcification, thickening, effusion, or cysts; and regional and global function assessment of the left and right ventricle (**Table 4.1**). Tracing of the left ventricular epicardial contour and the left ventricular cavity contour provides quantitative information about left ventricular wall motion as well as wall thickness and thickening.

Patency vs. occlusion of coronary artery bypass grafts can be accurately assessed by CT. However, the accuracy for detection of graft stenoses, in particular at the distal anastomosis, is reduced. Depiction of pulmonary vein anatomy may be important in many clinical situations (before and after electrophysiological testing or therapy).

Table 4.1 Main topics of interest

1. Frequently asked questions
Coronary calcium scoring for risk stratification
Anomalous coronary arteries
Coronary stenosis
Pulmonary embolism and aortic dissection
Cardiac masses and thrombi
Aortic aneurysm and dissection
Cardiac calcification (heart valves and pericardium)
Evaluation of bypass grafts (patency, stenosis, and age of occlusion)
Angiographic characterization of left and right internal mammarian artery

2. Future or seldomly asked questions
Influence of medical therapy (i.e., statins) on calcium score
Evaluation of coronary stents
Left and right ventricular volumes, ejections fraction, stroke volume, mass, and regional dyssynergy
Severity of aortic valve stenosis
Plaque characterization (plaque composition)
Coronary collaterals
Dilatation of superior and inferior vena cava and hepatic veins
Severity of mitral valve insufficiency
Possibility of grafting of distal coronary artery segments in case of proximal occlusion
Pulmonary veins before and after electrophysiological therapy (abnormalities, stenoses)

4.3 CT as a Screening Test: Indications in Asymptomatic Individuals?

Risk assessment in asymptomatic individuals is an unresolved issue of significant clinical importance: 88% of the patients with acute cardiac events were classified as low or intermediate-risk patients before, and 25–45% of the patients with acute myocardial infarction or acute cardiac death were asymptomatic before.

Only little information is available regarding the diagnostic accuracy of CT in predicting CAD in high-risk asymptomatic patient groups (i.e., diabetic patients). In asymptomatic patients with intermediate risk for CAD, noninvasive testing may be useful in providing more accurate risk assessment. However, head-to-head comparisons of different methods (stress echo, scintigraphy, stress MRI, and CT) are lacking, or only single-center results obtained in small numbers of patients are available. Negative stress tests have a high negative predictive value, with event rates below 1% within the next 5–10 years. The presence of coronary calcium is frequently associated with coronary atherosclerosis, and the amount of coronary calcium correlates with the "total coronary plaque burden" (except in the case of patients with chronic renal failure). The absence of coronary calcium virtually rules out coronary atherosclerosis and is associated with a very low risk of adverse coronary events.

Recent studies have shown that coronary calcium quantification is an independent predictor of adverse cardiac events and all-cause mortality. The European and other international societies on cardiovascular disease prevention state that "the calcium score is an important parameter to detect asymptomatic individuals at high risk for future cardiovascular events." However, calcium scanning cannot be recommended as a screening method for the unselected population, but it may play a role in individuals with intermediate risk, because a low calcium score may downgrade them to a low-risk group, or a high score may promote them to a high-risk group with the need for intensive risk-factor intervention.

4.4 Risk-Benefit of Cardiac CT: Economic and Biological Costs of Cardiac Imaging

Increased awareness of the economic, biological, and environmental costs of cardiac imaging will hopefully lead to greater appropriateness, wisdom, and prudence on the part of both the prescriber and the practitioner. The medical imaging market consists of several billion tests per year worldwide, with at least one-third being performed for cardiovascular indications. As each test incurs a cost and often involves a risk to the patient, we should consider every unnecessary and unjustifiable test one test too many. As clinical cardiologists, we want to know about the costs, risk, and radiation exposure associated with each available test. Radiation exposure is not a factor in echocardiography or MRI, but a sestamibi scan corresponds to 500 chest X-rays and a thallium scan to 1,150 chest X-rays. A recent study by Correia et al. showed that more intense use of tests involving ionizing radiation is not associated with a higher awareness of its risks among professionals. Physicians working in a high-tech, tertiary-care referral center were described as being forgetful of the environmental impact, biorisks, dose exposure, and legal restrictions associated with the ionizing exams they prescribed or performed. This situation is complicated by the fact that in some instances the use of obscure or nonstandardized terminology can make it difficult for researchers and clinicians to really understand the dose and risks associated with different procedures.

In cardiac imaging, if we assume the average cost (not charges) of echocardiography to be 1, the cost of a CT is 3.1, that of myocardial scintigraphy 3.27, and that of MRI 5.51. Recently, Dewey and Hamm demonstrated that, from the perspective of society, multislice CT coronary angiography is the most cost-effective modality for the diagnosis of CAD, up to a pretest likelihood of disease of 60%. Invasive coronary angiography remains the most cost-effective modality in patients with a rather high likelihood of CAD (at least 60%).

Recommended Reading

1. Amis ES, Jr., Butler PF, Applegate KE, et al. American College of Radiology white paper on radiation dose in medicine. J Am Coll Radiol 2007; 4:272–84
2. Bax JJ, Schuijf JD. Which role for multislice computed tomography in clinical cardiology? Am Heart J 2005; 149:960–1
3. Dewey M, Hamm B. Cost effectiveness of coronary angiography and calcium scoring using CT and stress MRI for diagnosis of coronary artery disease. Eur Radiol 2007; 17:1301–9
4. Dewey M, Teige F, Schnapauff D, et al. Noninvasive detection of coronary artery stenoses with multislice computed tomography or magnetic resonance imaging. Ann Intern Med 2006; 145:407–15
5. Picano E. Economic and biological costs of cardiac imaging. Cardiovasc Ultrasound 2005; 3:13

Clinical Indications

M. Dewey

5.1 Suspected Coronary Artery Disease 31
5.2 Other Appropriate Clinical Indications .. 31
5.3 Potential Clinical Indications 35
5.4 Currently No Clinical Indications 38
5.5 Patient Referral 38
    Recommended Reading 38

> **Abstract**
>
> The clinically most relevant indications for coronary CT angiography are presented.

5.1 Suspected Coronary Artery Disease

The most obvious indication for CT coronary angiography is to exclude coronary artery disease (CAD) in patients with a low-to-intermediate pretest likelihood of disease, which is defined as a likelihood of approximately 20–70% (**Fig. 5.1**). This group includes patients with inconclusive findings in previous stress tests and those presenting with atypical angina. On the one hand, patients with a higher pretest likelihood of CAD (>70%; e.g., with typical angina, risk factors, and a positive stress test) should not undergo coronary CT angiography as the first-line modality, because more patients in this subgroup will require subsequent conventional coronary angiography as the negative predictive value of CT is reduced (making a negative CT result less reliable). On the other hand, the positive predictive value is rather low in patients with a very low pretest likelihood of CAD (<20%; e.g., with non-anginal chest pain and a negative stress test), and the CT findings would lead to many unnecessary conventional coronary angiographies.

Thus, the preferred patient population for CT coronary angiography has a pretest likelihood of CAD of 20–70%. In **Tables 5.1–5.3**, patients with a pretest likelihood in this range are highlighted in blue. The markings in the tables make it easy to identify those patients who are most likely to benefit from coronary CT angiography and to simultaneously exclude others who should not undergo this test. These tables may also be helpful in increasing the cost-effectiveness of coronary CT angiography, as costly and unnecessary secondary examinations, which are more likely in very low (<20%) and high-likelihood patients (>70%), can potentially increase societal costs related to the diagnosis of CAD.

5.2 Other Appropriate Clinical Indications

Other justified indications for coronary CT angiography in addition to suspected CAD are summarized in **Table 5.4**. The quantitatively most important of these indications is imaging and follow-up of symptomatic patients with coronary artery bypass grafts (e.g., recurrent chest pain; Chap. 11). There is good evidence that CT allows highly accurate assessment of both the native coronaries and the bypass grafts in a single examination. However, the native coronary arteries in patients after bypass grafting are not as easily assessed as are the bypasses themselves, and only a few studies have addressed the combined reading of coronaries and bypasses. Thus, scientific evidence most strongly supports the use of MSCT for exclusion of CAD in patients with low-to-intermediate pretest likelihood (e.g., patients with suspected CAD and inconclusive findings and complaints).

The presence of coronary artery anomalies is also readily ruled out with CT, which is superior to magnetic resonance imaging (MRI) in depicting the distal parts of the coronaries and visualizing the entire course of anomalous vessels. Moreover, CT is well suited for follow-up of coronary aneurysms; however, in young patients, such as those with Kawasaki syndrome, MRI should be the first-line imaging tool because it does not involve radiation exposure, and there is no need for contrast agent administration.

CT is also highly accurate in analyzing global and regional cardiac function. MSCT has the crucial advantage that the images necessary for cardiac function analysis are inherently part of a standard coronary CT angiography, and no additional injection of contrast agent or radiation exposure is required. Therefore, because of the importance of global as well as regional cardiac function for the patient's prognosis and further management (Chap. 9), we strongly encourage the inclusion of cardiac function analysis in the reports of all patients undergoing coronary CT angiography. Nevertheless, because of the radiation exposure and the need for a contrast medium, CT is rarely indicated for analysis of cardiac function alone, but rather for use in combination with other clinical questions to be answered.

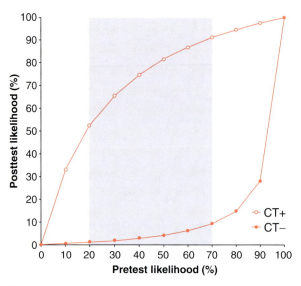

Fig. 5.1 The patient population with suspected CAD that is clinically most suitable for undergoing coronary CT angiography is highlighted in blue and has a pretest likelihood of disease of 20–70%. CT coronary angiography is very accurate in ruling out disease over a wide range of clinical presentations, as can be seen in the very low posttest likelihood after a negative CT (below 10% for pretest likelihoods of up to 70%). Thus, coronary CT angiography allows reliable exclusion of disease. However, patients with a likelihood of less than 20% may not benefit from noninvasive testing because of the very low positive predictive value in this group, which may lead to a rather high rate of unnecessary conventional coronary angiographies. This calculation, made according to the Bayes theorem, is based on the overall sensitivity and specificity of coronary CT angiography in patients with suspected CAD, as specified in Chap. 11

Table 5.1 Likelihood (in %) of CAD according to sex, age, and symptoms[a]

	Women				Men		
Age (years)	Nonanginal chest pain[b]	Atypical angina[c]	Typical angina[d]	Age (years)	Nonanginal chest pain[b]	Atypical angina[c]	Typical angina[d]
30–39	0.8	4	26	30–39	5	22	70
40–49	3	13	55	40–49	14	46	87
50–59	8	32	79	50–59	22	59	92
60–69	19	54	91	60–69	28	67	94

[a] The range of patients who are most likely to benefit from coronary CT angiography is highlighted in blue (those with a likelihood of 20–70%). In the 30- to 69-year age range, all men with atypical symptoms would be expected to benefit from CT, whereas women with atypical angina pectoris would be suitable candidates for coronary CT angiography only if they were older than 50 years of age. Modified from Diamond and Forrester, New Engl J Med 1979

[b] Only one of the three characteristics of angina pectoris is present (either retrosternal localization of pain, pain precipitated by exercise or decreased at rest, or on nitrate medication)

[c] Only two of the three characteristics of angina pectoris are present

[d] All of the three characteristics of angina pectoris are present

Table 5.2 Posttest likelihood (in %) of CAD in women after an electrocardiographic stress test (ST depression), according to age and symptoms[a]

ST depression (mm)	Age (years)	Women			
		Asymptomatic	Nonanginal chest pain[b]	Atypical angina[c]	Typical angina[d]
0–0.5	30–39	0.1	0.2	1	7
	40–49	0.2	0.7	3	22
	50–59	0.8	2	10	47
	60–69	2	5	21	69
0.5–1.0	30–39	0.3	0.7	4	24
	40–49	0.9	3	12	53
	50–59	3	8	31	78
	60–69	7	17	52	90
1.0–1.5	30–39	0.6	2	9	42
	40–49	2	6	25	72
	50–59	7	16	50	89
	60–69	15	33	72	95
1.5–2.0	30–39	1	3	16	59
	40–49	4	11	39	84
	50–59	12	28	67	94
	60–69	25	49	83	98
2–2.5	30–39	3	8	33	79
	40–49	10	24	63	93
	50–59	27	50	84	98
	60–69	47	72	93	99.1
> 2.5	30–39	11	24	63	93
	40–49	28	53	86	98
	50–59	56	78	95	99.3
	60–69	76	90	98	99.7

[a] The range of women who are most likely to benefit from coronary CT angiography is highlighted in blue (20–70%). Modified from Diamond and Forrester, New Engl J Med 1979

[b] Only one of the three characteristics of angina pectoris is present (either retrosternal localization of pain, pain precipitated by exercise or decreased at rest, or on nitrate medication)

[c] Only two of the three characteristics of angina pectoris are present

[d] All of the three characteristics of angina pectoris are present

Please note that 1.0 mm is equal to 0.1 mV

Table 5.3 Posttest likelihood (in %) of CAD in men after an electrocardiographic stress test (ST depression), according to age and symptoms[a]

ST depression (mm)	Age (years)	Men			
		Asymptomatic	Nonanginal chest pain[b]	Atypical angina[c]	Typical angina[d]
0–0.5	30–39	0.4	1	6	25
	40–49	1	4	16	61
	50–59	2	6	25	73
	60–69	3	8	32	79
0.5–1.0	30–39	2	5	21	68
	40–49	5	13	44	86
	50–59	9	20	57	91
	60–69	11	26	65	94
1.0–1.5	30–39	4	1	38	83
	40–49	11	26	64	94
	50–59	19	37	75	96
	60–69	23	45	81	97
1.5–2.0	30–39	8	19	55	91
	40–49	20	41	78	97
	50–59	31	53	86	98
	60–69	37	62	90	99
2.0–2.5	30–39	18	38	76	96
	40–49	39	65	91	99
	50–59	54	75	94	99.2
	60–69	61	81	96	99.5
> 2.5	30–39	43	68	92	99
	40–49	69	87	97	99.6
	50–59	81	91	98	99.8
	60–69	85	94	99	99.8

[a] The range of men who are most likely to benefit from coronary CT angiography is highlighted in blue (20–70%). Modified from Diamond and Forrester, New Engl J Med 1979

[b] Only one of the three characteristics of angina pectoris is present (either retrosternal localization of pain, pain precipitated by exercise or decreased at rest, or on nitrate medication)

[c] Only two of the three characteristics of angina pectoris are present

[d] All of the three characteristics of angina pectoris are present

Please note that 1.0 mm is equal to 0.1 mV

Table 5.4 Appropriate clinical indications for coronary CT angiography

	Pros	Cons
Exclusion of CAD in patients with low to intermediate pretest likelihood	High negative predictive value of CT Noninvasive CT is highly accepted by patients	Only little data available on possible advantages of CT over other modalities such as stress ECG, and on possible advantages for patient management
Patients with suspected CAD and inconclusive noninvasive test results	High negative predictive value of CT Noninvasive CT is highly accepted by patients	Only little data available on possible advantages for patient management
Follow-up of symptomatic patients with coronary artery bypasses	Reliable visualization of the entire bypass, including the proximal and distal anastomoses Noninvasive CT is highly accepted by patients	Only little data available on possible advantages for patient management Numerous studies, but in small patient populations
Exclusion of coronary artery anomalies and aneurysms	Excellent evaluation of the course of anomalous coronaries (malignant vs. benign) Unlike MRI, CT allows reliable visualization of the entire course of the vessel	Its competitor, MRI, is to be preferred, especially in younger patients, because it does not involve radiation exposure Unreliable in visualizing intracoronary collaterals
Analysis of global and regional cardiac function and valvular function[a]	CT has high spatial resolution[b] All data needed for functional analysis can be derived from CT coronary angiography without the need for an additional scan	Temporal resolution of CT is limited MRI and echocardiography are the established scientific and clinical gold standards

[a] Analysis of cardiac function is very fast and easy to perform using recent software tools, and because of its clinical importance, it should be performed and reported in every patient undergoing cardiac CT. In only rare cases there is a clinical indication for cardiac function analysis alone. Functional analysis is nearly always done as part of coronary CT angiography performed for other clinical indications

[b] CT performs better than echocardiography and cineventriculography

5.3 Potential Clinical Indications

There are also potential indications for coronary CT angiography, which we have summarized in **Table 5.5**. One such indication is in patients presenting with acute chest pain (without ST elevation) for which results of single-center studies are available. These studies have suggested that management of patients with acute chest pain might be streamlined with CT. However, these findings will have to be confirmed in larger, and particularly randomized, studies. If the results of such studies confirm the usefulness of performing immediate CT in patients presenting to the emergency department, then performing coronary CT angiography in these patients would be justified. In contrast, the so-called triple rule-out (to exclude coronary stenoses, pulmonary embolism, and aortic dissection) is still limited by the fact that no generally accepted scanning protocols are available, and the patient population that might benefit from such a comprehensive examination remains to be clearly defined (**Table 5.6**). Further larger studies investigating the benefit of CT in this respect are necessary before its general use can be considered.

CT coronary stent imaging is another potential clinical indication. However, the available evidence (Chap. 11) clearly indicates a reduced diagnostic accuracy in stents with a diameter of less than 3.5 mm. Also, because such stents represent 70–80% of all implanted coronary stents, in patients with more than two coronary stents the diagnostic accuracy will very likely be limited. Thus, there is no general indication for follow-up using currently available CT technology in patients after stent placement (**Table 5.5**). Also, the positive predictive value of CT is limited in coronary stent imaging (Chap. 11). The decision for or against CT should be made individually on the basis of the stent material and diameter; however, selected patients with low and stable heart rates can successfully be analyzed using CT angiography.

Table 5.5 Potential clinical indications for coronary CT angiography

	Pros	Cons
Acute chest pain without ST segment elevation	Reliable exclusion of CAD in these patients may be possible Patients may be discharged earlier or directly referred for bypass surgery[a]	There are as yet no results from studies in larger patient populations Unclear outcome benefit over established tests
Ruling out CAD prior to noncoronary cardiac surgery	Reliable exclusion of CAD in these patients may be possible Conventional coronary angiography may be avoided	There are as yet no results from studies in larger patient populations Unclear outcome benefit over established tests
Follow-up of patients with coronary artery stents	High negative predictive value for some stents Can be used for noninvasive follow-up	Evaluation of stents with an internal diameter < 3.5 mm is still limited Current CT technology does not provide functional information on blood flow direction
Prior to reoperative cardiac surgery	Important pathology (such as sternal wire near bypasses) and dimensions (e.g., distance of sternum to bypass) can be detected prior to operation	There are as yet no results from studies in larger patient populations
Suspected pericardial disease	Excellent depiction of calcified pericarditis ("armored heart") and pericardial effusion	CT provides only limited functional information MRI and echocardiography yield good results without radiation exposure

[a] Without the need for conventional coronary angiography

Table 5.6 Currently no clinical indications for coronary CT angiography

	Pros	Cons
Screening of asymptomatic individuals without abnormal findings in other noninvasive tests	May conceivably be more accurate than other noninvasive modalities in reliably excluding disease	The positive predictive value is unacceptably low in screening patients with a very low pretest likelihood of CAD (**Fig. 5.1**) Study results are not yet available
High pretest likelihood of CAD based on typical symptoms or positive results of other noninvasive tests	High negative predictive value	The negative predictive value is unacceptably low in patients with high pretest likelihood of CAD (**Fig. 5.1**) Study results are not yet available
Triple rule-out (to exclude coronary stenoses, pulmonary embolism, and aortic dissection)	Comprehensive examination	Generally accepted scanning protocols, and the target population remain to be defined No outcome studies
Analysis of myocardial viability and perfusion	CT has higher spatial resolution than MRI	Stress echocardiography and MRI have good clinical accuracy without involving radiation exposure Analysis of myocardial vitality and perfusion by CT requires an additional scan after coronary angiography

5.3 • Potential Clinical Indications

CHARITÉ

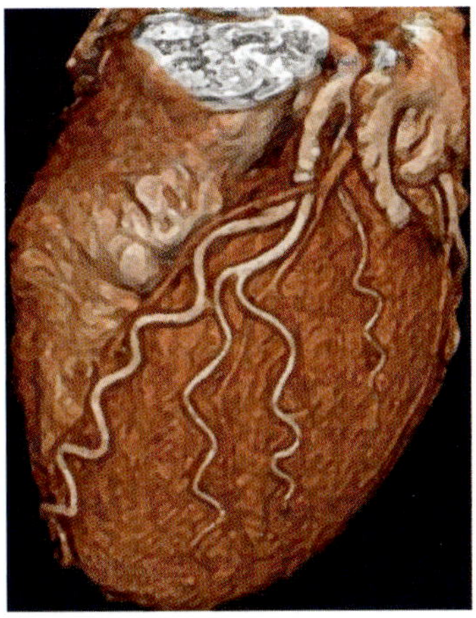

Referred by

Name: ....

Phone: ....

Address: ....

Referral for Coronary CT Angiography

Charité Campus Mitte   ○ **FAX:**
Dept. of Radiology   +49 (0)30/450 527 911
Charité platz 1
10117 Berlin, Germany

I request a **CT coronary angiography** for the following patient:
Last name: .... First name: .... D.O.B.:   .   .
Address: ....Phone: ....

Reason for exam: ○ Suspected CAD ○ Follow-up bypass ○ Follow-up stent ○ Other: ....
Indication/Question/Risk factors:
....
....

If the patient has undergone previous tests: Which? **(please attach reports)**
○ ECG ○ Stress ECG ○ Echo ○ Stress echo ○ Cardiac scintigraphy ○ MRI ○ CT

In patients with bypasses: No. of bypassess: .... Date of operation: ....
○ LIMA to ...... ○ RIMA to ...... No. of veins to: ○ LAD: ...... ○ LCX: ...... ○ RCA: ......○ Other: ....

Provision of the following information is **mandatory** in patients with stents to decide whether CT is reasonable:
No. of stents: ...... Stent diameter (mm): ..../......./......./........
Stent length (mm): ..../......./......./........ Stent site: ..../......./......./........

Did the patient have a conventional coronary angiography? Date :   .   .
Findings: ....

We ask for the following information so that we can exclude contraindications to CT:
Creatinine: .... ○ Hyperthyroidism (TSH: ....) ○ Allergic reaction to iodinated contrast agent
○ Irregular heart rate (e.g. atrial fibrillation): .... ○ Severe asthma (if high heart rate)
Please contact us by phone (+49 (0)30 450 527 133) if your patient has a contraindication or if you have further questions.

Fig. 5.2 Example of a referral form that can be used for coronary CT angiography

5.4 Currently No Clinical Indications

In our opinion, screening is definitely not an established clinical indication for coronary CT angiography at present (**Table 5.6**) because its predictive value for the presence of significant stenoses is too low in this patient population (**Fig. 5.1**). In contrast, the negative predictive value is very low in patients with typical symptoms and/or positive results of noninvasive tests (high pretest likelihood), so that CT is also not reliable enough to exclude coronary stenoses in this group.

Visualization and analysis of myocardial viability and perfusion is likewise not an accepted clinical indication for CT (**Table 5.6**). The main drawback of myocardial viability and perfusion imaging by CT is that extra scans with additional radiation exposure are necessary, whereas MRI yields excellent results without radiation exposure.

5.5 Patient Referral

We recommend using a special referral form, to be completed by physicians referring a patient for coronary CT angiography (**Fig. 5.2**). The information provided in the form makes it easier to decide whether the patient will benefit most from CT or another test. It also helps standardize and facilitate communication with referring physicians. Moreover, possible contraindications (Chap. 6) can be identified before an appointment is made, and the radiologist can choose in advance the most appropriate kind of coronary CT angiography (Chap. 7) to be performed in the patient (**Fig. 5.2**).

In summary, the decision as to whether there is a clinical indication for coronary CT angiography should always be made on an individual basis and should take into account the patient's pretest likelihood and possible contraindications.

Recommended Reading

1. Achenbach S. Computed tomography coronary angiography. J Am Coll Cardiol 2006; 48:1919–28
2. Cademartiri F, Schuijf JD, Pugliese F, et al. Usefulness of 64-slice multislice computed tomography coronary angiography to assess in-stent restenosis. J Am Coll Cardiol 2007; 49:2204–10
3. Cordeiro MA, Lima JA. Atherosclerotic plaque characterization by multidetector row computed tomography angiography. J Am Coll Cardiol 2006; 47:C40–C47
4. de Roos A, Kroft LJ, Bax JJ, Geleijns J. Applications of multislice computed tomography in coronary artery disease. J Magn Reson Imaging 2007; 26:14–22
5. Dewey M, Hamm B. CT Coronary angiography: Examination technique, clinical results, and outlook on future developments. Fortschr Röntgenstr 2007; 179:246–60
6. Dewey M, Müller M, Eddicks S, et al. Evaluation of global and regional left ventricular function with 16-slice computed tomography, biplane cineventriculography, and two-dimensional transthoracic echocardiography: Comparison with magnetic resonance imaging. J Am Coll Cardiol 2006; 48:2034–44
7. Dewey M, Teige F, Schnapauff D, et al. Noninvasive detection of coronary artery stenoses with multislice computed tomography or magnetic resonance imaging. Ann Intern Med 2006; 145:407–15
8. Diamond GA, Forrester JS. Analysis of probability as an aid in the clinical diagnosis of coronary-artery disease. N Engl J Med 1979; 300:1350–8
9. Ehara M, Kawai M, Surmely JF, et al. Diagnostic accuracy of coronary in-stent restenosis using 64-slice computed tomography: comparison with invasive coronary angiography. J Am Coll Cardiol 2007; 49:951–9
10. Feuchtner GM, Dichtl W, Friedrich GJ, et al. Multislice computed tomography for detection of patients with aortic valve stenosis and quantification of severity. J Am Coll Cardiol 2006; 47:1410–7
11. Feuchtner GM, Dichtl W, Schachner T, et al. Diagnostic performance of MDCT for detecting aortic valve regurgitation. AJR Am J Roentgenol 2006; 186:1676–81
12. Garcia MJ, Lessick J, Hoffmann MH. Accuracy of 16-row multidetector computed tomography for the assessment of coronary artery stenosis. JAMA 2006; 296:403–11
13. Gaspar T, Halon DA, Lewis BS, et al. Diagnosis of coronary in-stent restenosis with multidetector row spiral computed tomography. J Am Coll Cardiol 2005; 46:1573–9
14. Gasparovic H, Rybicki FJ, Millstine J, et al. Three dimensional computed tomographic imaging in planning the surgical approach for redo cardiac surgery after coronary revascularization. Eur J Cardiothorac Surg 2005; 28:244–9
15. Gilard M, Cornily JC, Pennec PY, et al. Assessment of coronary artery stents by 16 slice computed tomography. Heart 2006; 92:58–61
16. Hamon M, Biondi-Zoccai GG, Malagutti P, Agostoni P, Morello R, Valgimigli M. Diagnostic performance of multislice spiral computed tomography of coronary arteries as compared with conventional invasive coronary angiography: a meta-analysis. J Am Coll Cardiol 2006; 48:1896–910
17. Hamon M, Champ-Rigot L, Morello R, Riddell JW. Diagnostic accuracy of in-stent coronary restenosis detection with multislice spiral computed tomography: A meta-analysis. Eur Radiol 2008; 18:217–25
18. Hendel RC, Patel MR, Kramer CM, et al. ACCF/ACR/SCCT/SCMR/ASNC/NASCI/SCAI/SIR 2006 appropriateness criteria for cardiac computed tomography and cardiac magnetic resonance imaging. J Am Coll Cardiol 2006; 48:1475–97
19. Hoffmann MH, Shi H, Schmitz BL, et al. Noninvasive coronary angiography with multislice computed tomography. JAMA 2005; 293:2471–8
20. Hoffmann U, Pena AJ, Cury RC, et al. Cardiac CT in emergency department patients with acute chest pain. Radiographics 2006; 26:963–78; discussion 79–80
21. Jones CM, Athanasiou T, Dunne N, et al. Multi-detector computed tomography in coronary artery bypass graft assessment: A meta-analysis. Ann Thorac Surg 2007; 83:341–8
22. Leber AW, Johnson T, Becker A, et al. Diagnostic accuracy of dual-source multi-slice CT-coronary angiography in patients with an intermediate pretest likelihood for coronary artery disease. Eur Heart J 2007; 28:2354–60

23. Mahnken AH, Muhlenbruch G, Gunther RW, Wildberger JE. Cardiac CT: Coronary arteries and beyond. Eur Radiol 2007; 17:994–1008
24. Malagutti P, Nieman K, Meijboom WB, et al. Use of 64-slice CT in symptomatic patients after coronary bypass surgery: Evaluation of grafts and coronary arteries. Eur Heart J 2006; 28:1879–85
25. Martuscelli E, Romagnoli A, D'Eliseo A, et al. Evaluation of venous and arterial conduit patency by 16-slice spiral computed tomography. Circulation 2004; 110:3234–8
26. Meijboom WB, Mollet NR, Van Mieghem CA, et al. Pre-operative computed tomography coronary angiography to detect significant coronary artery disease in patients referred for cardiac valve surgery. J Am Coll Cardiol 2006; 48:1658–65
27. Meijboom WB, van Mieghem CA, Mollet NR, et al. 64-slice computed tomography coronary angiography in patients with high, intermediate, or low pretest probability of significant coronary artery disease. J Am Coll Cardiol 2007; 50:1469–75
28. Meyer TS, Martinoff S, Hadamitzky M, et al. Improved noninvasive assessment of coronary artery bypass grafts with 64-slice computed tomographic angiography in an unselected patient population. J Am Coll Cardiol 2007; 49:946–50
29. Mollet NR, Cademartiri F, Nieman K, et al. Multislice spiral computed tomography coronary angiography in patients with stable angina pectoris. J Am Coll Cardiol 2004; 43:2265–70
30. Poon M, Rubin GD, Achenbach S, et al. Consensus update on the appropriate usage of cardiac computed tomographic angiography. J Invasive Cardiol 2007; 19:484–90
31. Rixe J, Achenbach S, Ropers D, et al. Assessment of coronary artery stent restenosis by 64-slice multi-detector computed tomography. Eur Heart J 2006; 27:2567–72
32. Ropers U, Ropers D, Pflederer T, et al. Influence of heart rate on the diagnostic accuracy of dual-source computed tomography coronary angiography. J Am Coll Cardiol 2007; 50:2393–8
33. Schoepf UJ, Zwerner PL, Savino G, Herzog C, Kerl JM, Costello P. Coronary CT angiography. Radiology 2007; 244:48–63
34. Stillman AE, Oudkerk M, Ackerman M, et al. Use of multidetector computed tomography for the assessment of acute chest pain: A consensus statement of the North American Society of Cardiac Imaging and the European Society of Cardiac Radiology. Eur Radiol 2007; 17:2196–207
35. van der Vleuten PA, Willems TP, Gotte MJ, et al. Quantification of global left ventricular function: comparison of multidetector computed tomography and magnetic resonance imaging. A meta-analysis and review of the current literature. Acta Radiol 2006; 47:1049–57
36. Van Mieghem CA, Cademartiri F, Mollet NR, et al. Multislice spiral computed tomography for the evaluation of stent patency after left main coronary artery stenting: A comparison with conventional coronary angiography and intravascular ultrasound. Circulation 2006; 114:645–53
37. Weustink AC, Meijboom WB, Mollet NR, et al. Reliable high-speed coronary computed tomography in symptomatic patients. J Am Coll Cardiol 2007; 50:786–94

Patient Preparation

M. Dewey

6.1 Patient Information Sheets 41
6.2 General Information 41
6.3 Contraindications 44
     Recommended Reading 45

Abstract

Patient preparation is the key to success in coronary CT angiography, and the relevant aspects of this step are discussed in detail in this chapter.

6.1 Patient Information Sheets

As patient preparation is the cornerstone of a successful coronary CT angiography, a well-trained nurse, physician assistant, technician, or a physician (according to state and/or federal legal regulations) should discuss the entire procedure with the patient and obtain written informed consent. Patient education can be facilitated by sending the patient an information sheet and questionnaire before the appointment (**Figs. 6.1** and **6.2**). The information asked in the questionnaire also serves to verify the patient's clinical indication for coronary CT angiography and exclude possible clinical contraindications to the examination (Chap. 5).

6.2 General Information

The patient should be assured that CT is a noninvasive diagnostic procedure and that it does not take long to perform the examination. The short duration of the CT examination (about 15 min in the scanner room) and the comfortably wide and short gantry (in contrast to the narrow, claustrophobia-inducing bore in MRI) are major advantages of CT over MRI and should be stressed while talking to the patient. On the one hand, clearly explaining these aspects before the patient enters the scanner room reduces psychological stress and may relax the patient as well as reduce heart rate in some cases. On the other hand, the patient must also be given explicit information about the radiation exposure, which is the most important disadvantage of CT coronary angiography. As it does not mean much to a layperson that the effective exposure of a coronary CT exam is approximately 10–20 mSv, meaningful comparisons should be used, such as "the radiation exposure of coronary CT angiography is five to ten times the annual background radiation" or "the effective radiation dose of CT coronary angiography is the same as that of 100–200 chest X-rays." Especially in younger patients with a higher lifetime risk of cancer induced by CT, it is essential to carefully consider alternative imaging tests that might yield the same clinical information without radiation exposure.

Patients should know that a lower heart rate (associated with longer cardiac rest periods) improves image quality. Informing them about the entire procedure prevents inadvertent reactions to unexpected events that might increase their heart rate. Hence, patients should be informed that they might experience a sensation of warmth when the contrast medium is injected and should also be told beforehand about the expected duration and number of breath-hold periods. Patients who are aware that the target structures are just a few millimeters in size will better understand that any motion during the breath-hold periods may severely degrade the images and may even result in a nondiagnostic scan. They also need to be informed that they should hold their breath after submaximal inspiration (ca. 75% of maximum inspiration), a maneuver that should be taught either prior to the examination or during scanning as part of the training related to the breath-hold commands (Chap. 7).

CHARITÉ

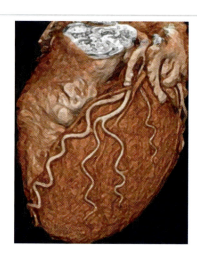

Patient Information
CT Coronary Angiography

Dear Ms./Mr. ....,

Your doctor has referred you for an examination of your heart vessels (coronary arteries) to look for narrowings (stenoses) and deposits (plaques). The examination is performed on a computed tomography (CT) scanner. CT identifies stenoses and plaques in the coronary arteries with a reliability of over 90% and we expect that the information gained by the examination will help improve your further treatment.

You should fast for four hours before the examination (most importantly, you should not drink coffee or tea) and should continue to take your usual medications. If you take the antidiabetic drug called metformin, you must stop taking this medication for 48 hours after the test.

Please carefully complete the questionnaire provided with this information sheet (see **Figure 6.2**). The details about your symptoms and other tests that you have had in the past will help us make the correct diagnosis by CT. A written report of the CT findings will be sent to your doctor after the examination.

Please send the completed form to the address or fax number given below or bring it along when you come in for your examination on day: .... at: ....

Address:
Charité
Institut für Radiologie, CT
Luisenstr. 68 (Hochhaus)
10117 Berlin

FAX No.:
+49 (0)30/450 527 911

Phone:
+49 (0)30/450 527 133

Most patients with one of the following conditions cannot undergo a CT scan of the heart:
1. Irregular heart beat (e.g., atrial fibrillation)
2. Severe bronchial asthma (if high heart rate is present)
3. Intake of certain erectile dysfunction pills (e.g., Viagra)
4. Reduced kidney function (creatinine level > 1.5 – 2.0 mg/dl)
5. Allergic reactions to X-ray contrast media
6. Manifest overactivity of the thyroid (hyperthyroidism)

If one of these conditions applies in your case, please contact us before the examination

Fig. 6.1 Example of an information sheet that is sent out to the patient prior to the examination. Patients are asked to inform us in case contraindications to coronary CT angiography might be present that have been overlooked during the prior referral procedure (Chap. 5)

Patient Questionnaire

Name: .... Address: .... Phone No.: ....

FAX: .... Email: ....@..............................

1. **D.O.B.**: . . . **Height**: . m/inches **Weight**: .... kg/pounds **male** ○ **female** ○
2. Do you have **pain** in the chest? yes ○ no ○, If yes, please describe the location and type of pain:

   ....

   Does the pain increase when you **exercise**? yes ○ no ○ How long does the pain last? ....

   Does the pain decrease **at rest or after nitro spray**? yes ○ no ○
3. Do you **smoke**? yes ○ no ○ If yes, for how long? .... years, how many cigarettes per day? ......
4. Did you **smoke**? yes ○ no ○ If yes, for how long? .... years, how many cigarettes per day? ......
5. Do you have **high blood lipid levels** (hyperlipidemia)? yes ○ no ○

   Total cholesterol: ....(p≥200 mg/dl) **LDL**: ...... (p≥120 mg/dl) **TG**: ......(p≥200mg/dl)
6. Do you take **statins** or other drugs to lower cholesterol? yes ○ no ○ - for how long? .... years
7. Do you have **high blood sugar** (diabetes mellitus)? yes ○ no ○
8. Do you have **high blood pressure** (hypertension)? yes ○ no ○
9. Do you take **beta blockers** to lower blood pressure? yes ○ no ○ - for how long? .... years
10. Have you had a **heart attack** (myocardial infarction)? yes ○ no ○, If yes, please bring the report with you.
11. Do you have **stents** that keep the heart vessels open? yes ○ no ○, If yes, please bring the report with you.
12. Have you had **widening of a vessel** with a catheter? yes ○ no ○, If yes, please bring the report with you.
13. Do you have any cardiac **bypasses**? yes ○ no ○, If yes, please bring the report with you.
14. Have you had an **electrocardiogram** (ECG)? yes ○ no ○, If yes, please bring the report with you.
15. Have you had an **exercise (treadmill) ECG**? yes ○ no ○, If yes, please bring the report with you.
16. Have you had an **echocardiogram**? yes ○ no ○, If yes, please bring the report with you.
17. Have you had a **stress echocardiogram**? yes ○ no ○, If yes, please bring the report with you.
18. Have you had **myocardial scintigraphy**? yes ○ no ○, If yes, please bring the report with you.
19. Have you had a **cardiac catheter examination**? yes ○ no ○, If yes, please bring the report(s) with you.
20. Have you had a **CT scan/MRI** of the heart? yes ○ no ○, If yes, please bring the reports with you.
21. Which **medications** are you taking? Please list, **with doses**:

   - ....   - ....

   - ....   - ....

   - ....   - ....

Fig. 6.2 Example of a medical history questionnaire that is also sent out to the patient prior to the examination. This questionnaire elicits information about the patient's entire cardiovascular medical history and is very valuable for diagnostic procedures in the outpatient setting

The submaximum depth of inspiration is important, because maximal inspiration may increase intrathoracic pressure (Valsava maneuver) and reduce inflow of the contrast medium.

The length of the breath-hold periods varies between 8 and 30 s, depending on the scanner used and the examination performed. Breath-hold training on the scanner table is therefore also important to determine whether a patient is able to hold his or her breath for the required duration, or whether oxygen administration is needed to improve compliance. Preoxygenation is rarely required when the examination is performed on a 64-slice CT scanner, with scan times of only 8–12 s for coronary CT angiography.

6.3 Contraindications

When informing the patient about coronary CT angiography, the examiner should make sure that the patient is in sinus rhythm. This assessment is most easily accomplished by feeling the radial pulse when meeting the patient. In the case of patients with atrial fibrillation or frequent extrasystoles (at least one or two within the expected breath-hold period), the per-patient diagnostic accuracy is still unsatisfactory; for this reason, it is advisable that the examination be performed at a later time, for example after medical or electrical cardioversion.

At the same time, the patient should also be questioned about general contraindications to contrast agents (**List 6.1**), as well as contraindications to nitroglycerin (**List 6.2**) and beta blockers (**List 6.3**). The considerable radiation exposure involved (about 10–20 mSv) precludes coronary CT angiography in young and pregnant women. It is usually safe to administer nitroglycerin and/or beta blockers for the CT scan to patients who are taking these two medications on a regular basis without problems. Whether CT can be performed without nitroglycerin and/or beta blocker administration in patients with contraindications must be decided on an individual basis and depends on the clinical question and the patient's heart rate. It is generally desirable to administer nitroglycerin because of the beneficial vasodilatory effect. The CT scan should be postponed in patients who have taken phosphodiesterase inhibitors within the 24 h preceding the planned examination (**List 6.2**).

List 6.1. Contraindications to iodinated contrast agents

1. Renal insufficiency (creatinine level > 1.5–2.0 mg/dl, absolute contraindication unless evidence-based measures to prevent contrast-induced nephropathy can be taken)
2. Intake of metformin-containing medications (metformin needs to be discontinued for 48 h after contrast injection)[a]
3. Prior allergic reactions to iodinated contrast agents (switching to a different contrast agent and antiallergic premedication may enable imaging in those patients)
4. Manifest hyperthyroidism

[a] In patients with abnormal renal function, metformin also needs to be discontinued for 48 h prior to elective examinations, according to the ESUR guideline

---

List 6.2. Contraindications to nitroglycerin

1. Intake of phosphodiesterase inhibitors (such as sildenafil, tadalafil, and vardenafil)
2. Arterial hypotension (systolic blood pressure below 100 mm Hg)
3. Severe aortic stenosis
4. Hypertrophic obstructive cardiomyopathy
5. Nitroglycerin intolerance (e.g., severe headache)

List 6.3. Contraindications to beta blockers

1. Severe asthma
2. Severe obstructive lung disease
3. Bradycardia (below 50 beats per min)
4. Second or third degree atrioventricular block
5. Beta blocker intolerance (e.g., psoriasis)

Recommended Reading

1. Achenbach S. Computed tomography coronary angiography. J Am Coll Cardiol 2006; 48:1919–28
2. Achenbach S, Rost C, Ropers D, Pflederer T, von Erffa J, Daniel WG. Non-invasive coronary angiography: current status and perspectives. Dtsch Med Wochenschr 2007; 132:750–6
3. Dewey M, Hamm B. CT Coronary angiography: examination technique, clinical results, and outlook on future developments. Fortschr Röntgenstr 2007; 179:246–60
4. Dewey M, Hoffmann H, Hamm B. Multislice CT coronary angiography: effect of sublingual nitroglycerine on the diameter of coronary arteries. Fortschr Röntgenstr 2006; 178:600–04
5. Einstein AJ, Henzlova MJ, Rajagopalan S. Estimating risk of cancer associated with radiation exposure from 64-slice computed tomography coronary angiography. JAMA 2007; 298:317–23
6. Hoffmann U, Ferencik M, Cury RC, Pena AJ. Coronary CT angiography. J Nucl Med 2006; 47:797–806
7. Pannu HK, Alvarez W, Jr., Fishman EK. Beta-blockers for cardiac CT: a primer for the radiologist. AJR Am J Roentgenol 2006; 186: S341–5
8. Schoepf UJ, Zwerner PL, Savino G, Herzog C, Kerl JM, Costello P. Coronary CT angiography. Radiology 2007; 244: 48–63
9. Schönenberger E, Schnapauff D, Teige F, Laule M, Hamm B, Dewey M. Patient acceptance of noninvasive and invasive coronary angiography. PLoS ONE 2007; 2:e246
10. Weigold WG. Coronary CT angiography: insights into patient preparation and scanning. Tech Vasc Interv Radiol 2006; 9:205–9

The ESUR guideline on contrast media can be accessed at: http://www.esur.org/ESUR_Guidelines.6.0.html

Examination and Reconstruction

M. Dewey

7.1 Examination 47
7.1.1 Calcium Scoring 47
7.1.2 Positioning and ECG 48
7.1.3 Nitroglycerin 49
7.1.4 Beta Blockade 50
7.1.5 Planning the Scan 51
7.1.6 Breath-hold Training 53
7.1.7 Scanning Parameters 54
7.1.8 Contrast Agent 54
7.1.9 Starting the Scan 56
7.1.10 After the Scan 57
7.2 Reconstruction 57
7.2.1 Slice Thickness and Fields of View 58
7.2.2 Temporal Resolution and the Cardiac Reconstruction Phase 58
Recommended Reading 64

Abstract

In this chapter, the examination-related procedures are described.

The steps involved in coronary CT angiography are summarized in **List 7.1**. The entire examination procedure takes approximately 15–20 min.

> **List 7.1. Steps in performing coronary CT angiography**
>
> 1. Reassure the patient that the examination will be short and uncomplicated – consider oral beta blockers
> 2. Place the patient in a comfortable position
> 3. Place ECG electrodes to obtain good R-wave signals
> 4. Check heart rate and rhythm – consider injecting beta blockers
> 5. Plan scan range, and adjust scan and contrast agent parameters individually
> 6. Administer nitroglycerin sublingually
> 7. Provide breath-hold training
> 8. Repeat beta blocker injection if necessary
> 9. Inject the contrast agent – adjust scan delay individually
> 10. Perform the scan, and make sure that the patient is feeling fine afterward

7.1 Examination

The CT examination should be performed in a calm and comfortable atmosphere (e.g., lights should be dimmed, and the staff should speak quietly), avoiding anything that might affect the patient's heart rate, because a constant rate is crucial for image quality and diagnostic accuracy in coronary CT angiography. Patients should likewise avoid anything that can increase their heart rate, such as talking during the scan or moving too much.

7.1.1 Calcium Scoring

Unlike CT coronary angiography, coronary calcium scoring is always performed by using prospective triggering with 3-mm slice collimation without contrast administration and can help reduce radiation exposure by allowing exact determination of the scan range required for subsequent CT coronary angiography (from about 1 cm above to 1 cm below the coronaries). The clinical benefit of calcium scoring is not in detecting or ruling out coronary artery disease, but in risk stratification of individual patients. Combined coronary calcium scoring and angiography can be easily performed, and it prolongs the examination by only 3–5 min.

However, in patients with low-to-intermediate pretest likelihood of coronary artery disease, calcium scoring should not be performed alone, since angiography will demonstrate significant coronary stenoses in a considerable number of patients without coronary calcium or a low coronary calcium score. Very high calcium scores (above 400 or 600) are considered by some groups to preclude reliable reading of coronary CT angiography and may be used as a gatekeeper prior to noninvasive angiography. This approach, however, requires calculating or estimating the score during the examination and may reduce workflow. In our experience, neither image quality nor diagnostic accuracy is significantly reduced in patients with somewhat higher calcium scores, and patients with a 20–70% pretest likelihood of coronary disease only rarely have very high calcium scores. Therefore, we do not routinely perform calcium scoring in our patients with low-to-intermediate pretest likelihood of coronary artery disease. To sum up, the decision whether to perform coronary CT angiography alone or in combination with calcium scoring largely depends on the local situation and the individual patient's needs.

7.1.2 Positioning and ECG

Once the patient has been placed on the table in the supine position with the arms above the head (**Fig. 7.1**), he or she should not move, in order to ensure that the planned scan region matches the region actually scanned and that the entire coronary tree is imaged (**Fig. 7.2**). Spatial resolution is highest in the center of the scan field, which is why the patient should be shifted slightly to the right side of the table, so that the heart is as close to the center as possible (**Fig. 7.1**). The ECG electrodes should be placed so that they do not disturb the patient (**Fig. 7.1**), while ensuring optimal identification of R-wave signals (**Fig. 7.3**). The optimal electrode position is as close as possible to the heart but outside the anatomic scan field (**Fig. 7.4**), in order to avoid artifacts. If the electrodes are too far away from the chest (e.g., near the biceps or deltoid muscles), involuntary muscle shivering may be superimposed on the cardiac electrical activity (**Fig. 7.5**).

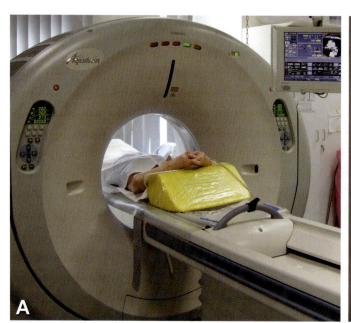
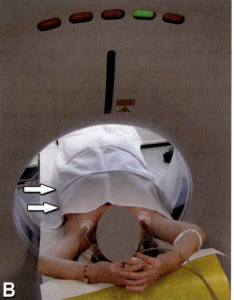

Fig. 7.1 Patient positioning for cardiac CT. Examining the patient feet-first (**Panel A**) has the advantage of providing better access to the patient than with head-first positioning. The arms are comfortably placed above the head to improve penetration of the chest by the X-rays, thereby reducing artifacts and radiation exposure. The patient is placed in an offset position, slightly to the right side of the table (*arrows*, **Panel B**), to ensure that the heart is as close as possible to the center of the scan field. ECG electrodes are attached in the area of the supraclavicular fossa after the patient has elevated his or her arms. The ECG electrodes should not be attached near the biceps or deltoid muscles, in order to minimize the effects of muscle tremor on the ECG (**Fig. 7.5**)

7.1 • Examination

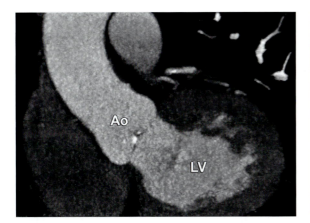

Fig. 7.2 Motion of the patient between planning of the scan and the actual scan resulted in a scan range that extended too far cranially, and therefore the caudal portions of the heart were missed. Oblique coronal maximum-intensity projection in the left ventricular outflow tract view. *Ao* aorta; *LV* left ventricle

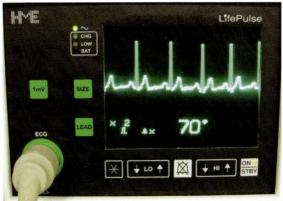

Fig. 7.3 ECG monitor with regular ECG and sufficiently high R waves for gating of the examination. However, heart rate reduction using beta blockade should be considered

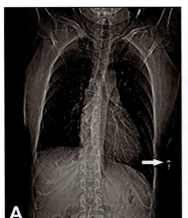 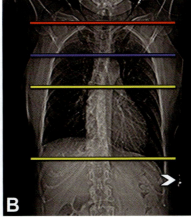 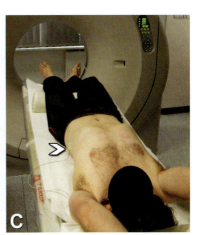

Fig. 7.4 Positioning of ECG leads and planning of the scan. A typical anterior scanogram (**Panel A**) with a too-high electrode (*arrow*) on the left side of the chest, which can lead to artifacts over the cardiac structures. Such artifacts can be easily avoided by lower placement of the electrode (*arrowhead* in **Panels B** and **C**). The typical anatomic scan range for patients with suspected or known coronary artery disease is indicated by the *yellow lines* and extends from above the left atrium to immediately below the heart (**Panel B**). Because of the high effective dose, the scan range should be as short as reasonably achievable. For imaging of venous (*blue line*) or internal mammary artery bypass grafts (*red line*), the beginning of the scan range needs to be extended (**Panel B**)

7.1.3 Nitroglycerin

Sublingual nitroglycerin administration increases the diameter of the coronary arteries (**Fig. 7.6**) and therefore facilitates image interpretation and comparability of the results (percent diameter stenosis) with those of cardiac catheter examination (which is often performed with intracoronary nitroglycerin administration). The onset of action of sublingual nitroglycerin spray (**Fig. 7.7A**) is about 10–20 s after administration, and its effect lasts for about 10–30 min. Patients should be given two to three sprays of sublingual nitroglycerin (corresponding to a dose of about 0.8–1.2 mg). Complications of nitroglycerin administration include tachycardia and hypotension (which may cause headaches). Relevant reflex tachycardia is rare, and this unlikely event should not prevent physicians from taking advantage of the beneficial vasodilatory effect of nitroglycerin (**Fig. 7.6**).

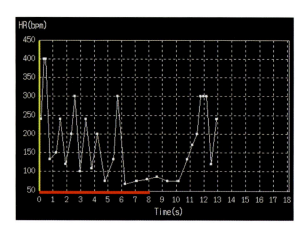

Fig. 7.5 Unconscious muscle shivering led to a highly variable (between 60 and 400 beats per min) and unreliable heart rate recording. Covering the patient with a blanket will reduce shivering, and the ECG will very likely become normal

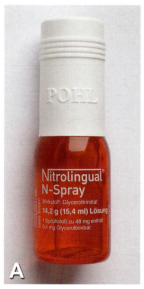 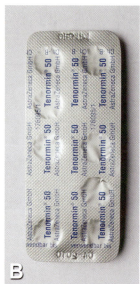

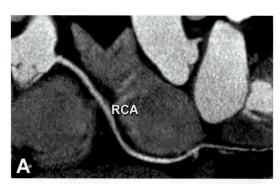

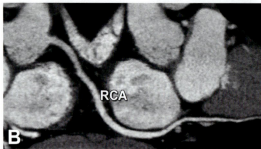

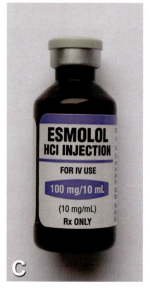 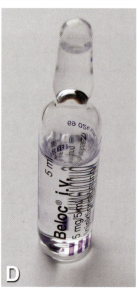

Fig. 7.6 Effect of sublingual nitroglycerin on the coronary vessel diameters. Curved multiplanar reformation of the right coronary artery (RCA) in a patient who underwent coronary CT angiography without (**Panel A**) and after sublingual nitroglycerin (**Panel B**). Nitroglycerin administration leads to a relevant increase in the coronary diameter (on average 12–21%), which also improves visibility of the distal vessel segments

Fig. 7.7 Drugs for premedication in patients undergoing coronary CT. Sublingual nitroglycerin (**Panel A**) increases coronary vessel diameters and facilitate comparison of the findings to conventional coronary angiography. Oral (**Panel B**, metoprolol or atenolol) and/or intravenous beta blockade (**Panels C** and **D**, esmolol or metoprolol) is important to reduce heart rate in order to improve image quality and increase diagnostic accuracy as much as possible

7.1.4 Beta Blockade

The heart rate can be reduced (**Fig. 7.8**) by oral administration of a beta blocker about 1 h before CT scanning (e.g., 50 mg atenolol, **Fig. 7.7B**), or intravenous administration of an agent with rapid onset of action and shorter duration of action (e.g., esmolol at a dose of 25–50 mg min^{-1} [0.5 mg kg^{-1} bodyweight per min], **Fig. 7.7C**; or metoprolol at 2.5–5 mg min^{-1}, **Fig. 7.7D**) with the patient on the table. All intravenous beta blockers should be injected slowly, and

7.1 · Examination

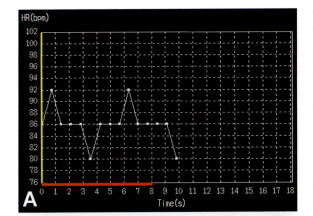
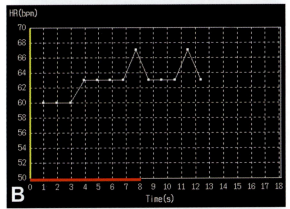
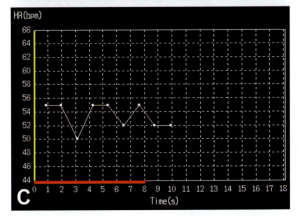

Fig. 7.8 Heart rate reduction using intravenous beta blockade. The patient (90 kg) had an initial heart rate of 80–92 beats per min during breath-hold training (**Panel A**). An initial dose of 10 mg metoprolol (equivalent to approximately 100 mg esmolol) reduced the heart rate to 60–67 beats per min (**Panel B**). After a second injection of 10 mg metoprolol, the patient's heart rate was adequately reduced to 50–55 beats per min during the final breath-hold training period (**Panel C**). Following contrast injection, the heart rate remained stable at 55 beats per min. In this case, the dose of intravenous beta blockers might have been reduced if oral beta blockers had been administered before the patient entered the scanner room

the examiner must wait and see how the patient reacts to the initial dose (e.g., 20–30 mg of esmolol) before determining the further injection protocol. The onset of action of esmolol is approximately 2–5 min, and the half-life is only 9–10 min. Therefore, a lower risk of complications such as bradycardia can be expected with intravenous beta blockade, while oral beta blockers tend to lower heart rate more markedly. A combination of oral and intravenous beta blockers is also effective.

In our experience, a resting heart rate of 65–70 beats per min is a good threshold above which to give intravenous beta blockers. Up to this threshold, good image quality can be achieved using adaptive multisegment reconstruction and dual-source CT. If these two techniques for improving spatial resolution are not available, lower thresholds may be considered (about 55–60 beats per min). In patients with heart rates of more than 80 beats per min, more effective heart rate reduction can be achieved by additional oral beta blockade. However, in general, beta blockers should be administered in accordance with local practice and guidelines where applicable. Note that atropine must be available as an antidote whenever beta blockers are given. Complications of beta blockers are bradycardia, hypotension, and acute asthmatic episodes. The foremost measure to alleviate the initial symptoms of bradicardia and hypotension is to elevate the patient's legs. Serious complications of beta blockers are very rare and, in patients with higher heart rates, should not prevent us from making use of the positive effects of beta blockers in terms of improved image quality and diagnostic accuracy. In case of an insufficient effect of beta blockade, intravenous conscious sedation (e.g., 1 mg of midazolam or lorazepam) is an alternative to slow the patient's heart rate.

7.1.5 Planning the Scan

When a CT scan is performed for suspected coronary disease or follow-up of coronary artery stents, the scan range extends from above the left atrium to immediately below the heart (**Figs. 7.4** and **7.9**). As 1 cm of a helical scan is equal to an effective dose of 1–2 mSv, every effort should be made to limit the scan range as much as possible. For imaging of the ascending aorta or the aortic and/or pulmonic valve, the start of the scan range needs to be extended above the aortic arch (**Fig. 7.4**). This scan range is also sufficient for patients who have undergone sole venous coronary bypass grafting, whereas in patients with left or right internal mammary artery grafts, the scan should start approximately in the middle of the clavicle (**Fig. 7.4**) to include the full length of these grafts.

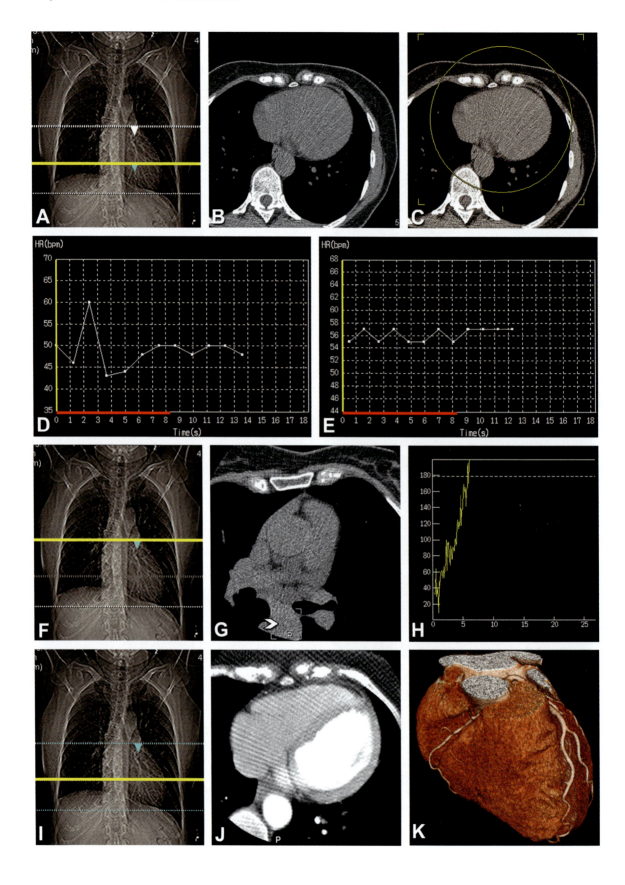

These different scan lengths highlight the importance of taking into account clinical information about previous treatments and diagnostic tests to tailor the examination to the individual patient's needs.

The scan field of view (axial extension of the radiated area) should be as small as possible to reduce the radiation exposure and, most important, to increase the spatial resolution (since small focus spots are used). We use, for instance, 320-mm scan fields of view (medium size) for coronary imaging, which reduces radiation exposure by 20–25% when compared with large scan fields of view (**Fig. 7.9**). The scan field of view needs to be differentiated from the smaller reconstruction field of view, which determines the size of the images to which the standard 512×512 CT matrix is applied. If the scanner allows the determination of this reconstruction field of view during the scanning procedure, it is clearly advisable to do so (**Fig. 7.9**), as this precaution will avoid potential mistakes, such as forgetting to reduce the reconstruction field of view afterward and reconstructing the coronary images on large fields of view.

7.1.6 Breath-hold Training

Temporal resolution can be improved by testing the patient's heart rate before the examination using the same breathing instructions ("Please breathe in and then hold your breath") as during the actual scan (**Fig. 7.9**). The information on the individual patient's heart rate range during the trial breath-hold can be used on some scanners to automatically adjust scan parameters such as pitch and gantry rotation time to the individual heart rate and heart rate variability. Even more importantly, breath-hold training ensures that a patient can actually hold his or her breath as long as necessary for the scan (**Fig. 7.10**). Heart rate variability during breath-hold training should be less than 10% (**Fig. 7.9**), because greater variability will degrade image quality. Breath-hold training is also a good opportunity to remind the patient that scanning

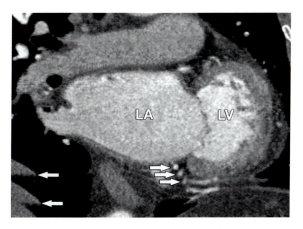

Fig. 7.10 Breathing-related motion artifacts leading to multiple visualizations of the right coronary artery and diaphragm and degraded images of the caudal portions of the heart (*arrows*). Such artifacts can be avoided in most patients by breath-hold training to ensure that the patient can hold his or her breath as long as is required for scanning. If the patient is unable to do so, breath-hold capacity can be improved by preoxygenation. *LA* left atrium; *LV* left ventricle

Fig. 7.9 Planning and conducting the scan. The scan range for a typical coronary CT extends from above the left atrium to immediately below the heart (*dotted lines* in **Panel A**). We then perform a single axial scan at the level of the largest diameter of the heart (**Panel B**), which is indicated by a *yellow line* in **Panel A**. We use this axial image to determine the 180–200 mm reconstruction field of view (*yellow circular region* in **Panel C**) to make optimal use of the maximum resolution provided by CT scanners (10 line pairs per cm). Breath-hold training not only familiarizes the patient with the breathing instructions for the actual coronary scans but also allows monitoring of heart rate and variability during this period (**Panel D**). If the heart rate variability is above 10% (43–60 beats per min), as shown in **Panel D**, either further relaxation of the patient or beta blockade is necessary to reduce the RR interval variability to less than 10%, as shown in **Panel E** (55–57 beats per min). By obtaining another axial scan at the level of the planned beginning of the helical coronary acquisition (**Panel F**), we can make sure that no coronary vessels are visible on this axial image (**Panel G**) that might not be included in the planned scan region. Alternatively, the unenhanced calcium scan can be used to define the start and end of the coronary scan. This axial image (**Panel G**) is also used to define a circular region of interest (*arrowhead*) in the descending aorta. This region of interest is subsequently used to track the arrival of the contrast agent bolus (**Panel H**) and to start the helical scan at a threshold of 180 Hounsfield units. Once the threshold has been reached, a simple, 5-s breathing instruction is given ("Please breathe in and then hold your breath"). The helical scan is then started with a delay of 3 s, to allow the heart to return to normal after inspiration. During the subsequent helical acquisition, the moving position of the online images is indicated by a *yellow line* on the scanogram (**Panel I**). These online images (**Panel J**, in this case showing an example at the level of the largest diameter of the heart) can be used to stop the acquisition once the caudal border of the heart has been reached, in order to reduce radiation as much as possible. The results of this coronary CT angiography are shown in **Panel K**

is not performed at full inspiration but at about 75% of maximum inspiration, because the increased intrathoracic pressure at full inspiration (Valsalva maneuver) might reduce inflow of the contrast agent.

7.1.7 Scanning Parameters

Tube current should be adjusted to the patient's body weight to ensure a constant high image quality regardless of body mass, while keeping the effective radiation dose to a minimum (**Table 7.1** and **Fig. 7.11**). The effective dose can be reduced most effectively by choosing the smallest possible scan range, since a range of about 1 cm corresponds to the effective radiation dose of 5–10 mammographies (each an effective dose of approximately 0.2 mSv). A further significant reduction (of 10–40%) can be achieved by ECG-gated tube current modulation. Nevertheless, this technique should only be used in patients with slow heart rates (<60 beats per min) and low heart rate variability, to avoid reduction of image quality. Tube current modulation resulting in much noisier systolic images might limit the application of regional and global (semi)automatic cardiac function analysis tools and is not recommended in these cases.

7.1.8 Contrast Agent

The flow of contrast agent, and thus its amount, should also be adjusted to the patient's body weight (**Table 7.2**) in order to compensate for the greater attenuation of X-rays in heavier patients and to achieve comparable contrast between the contrast-filled coronary lumen and the surrounding tissue over a wide range of body weights (**Table 7.2**). When coronary artery stents are being imaged, a higher density in the vessel lumen is beneficial, whereas for coronary plaque imaging, the density should not be too high (to avoid influencing of plaque density values, and potentially also plaque volumes). Thus, contrast agent flow may also have to be adapted to reflect the clinical question to be answered by the coronary CT angiography.

Biphasic injection of the contrast agent followed by a saline flush (using a dual-head injector) results in a more compact contrast bolus in the heart and ensures that the right ventricle and atrium are no longer filled with contrast when the coronary helical scan is started with an adequate delay. Ensuring this emptying of the ventricle and atrium significantly reduces the likelihood of streak artifacts arising from the right cardiac chambers, which can otherwise severely degrade the capacity to assess the right coronary artery. This simple dual bolus of contrast agent followed by saline is sufficient for coronary artery imaging. Because of the very low density in the right cardiac chambers, however, the septal wall might not be easily discernible, making it difficult to evaluate both regional and global left and right ventricular function. Thus, whenever cardiac function assessment is pivotal, two injection protocols can be used to improve the images: (1) dual-phase injection (e.g., 4 ml s^{-1} for 80% of the contrast agent, and 2 ml s^{-1} for the rest) followed by saline, or (2) injection of a mixture of contrast agent and saline as the second phase. In most "rule out coronary disease" patients, however, such sophisticated contrast agent injection techniques are not a must, and simple contrast agent administration with a saline flush is sufficient.

What is clearly more important than these issues is that at least a 20-gauge intravenous line is used for contrast agent injection. The right cubital veins are clearly preferable over the left side or hand veins, because the distance to the cardiac chambers is shortest this way and the contrast bolus is the least diluted. Moreover, using the right cubital vein is preferable because this approach avoids problems with streak artifacts from contrast agent in the left subclavian vein that might obscure the most common arterial bypass graft (left internal mammary artery).

Another area of concern is how to estimate and standardize the contrast agent amount that is injected for coronary CT angiography. The following formula can be used to calculate the amount of contrast agent for CT angiography on a 64-row scanner according to the individual helical scan duration:

Table 7.1 Scanner settings for CT coronary angiography

Body weight	kV	mA Pitch of 0.2 to <0.225^a	mA Pitch of ≥0.225
<60 kg (<132 lb)	120	300	300
60–80 kg (132–176 lb)	120	340	360
>80 kg (>176 lb)	120	360	400

^{a} The pitch can be adjusted according to the heart rate and heart rate variability during breath-hold training (see Chap. 7.1.6). The mA settings above are valid for Toshiba's Aquilion 64 scanner only. Optimal mA settings may be different on other scanners (Chap. 8). As a general rule, the mA should always be reduced in patients with lower body weight or body mass index and increased in heavier patients. An increase in kV (e.g., to 140) may be considered in very heavy patients (above 100 or 120 kg)

7.1 · Examination

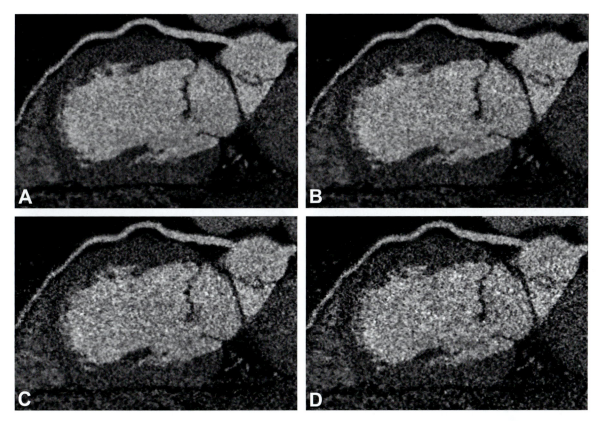

Fig. 7.11 Effect of tube current on image quality. Curved multiplanar reformations along the left anterior descending coronary artery in a patient with a body weight of 110 kg and a body-mass index of 32. The scan was acquired with a mA of 360 and is shown in **Panel A**. Using the raw data for this patient, we simulated (**Panels B–D**) what the images would look like with lower mA settings (performed in cooperation with Toshiba; Okumura-san and Noshi-san). These panels represent mA settings of 300 (**Panel B**), 250 (**Panel C**), and 200 (**Panel D**). Already at 300 mA (**Panel B**), the curved multiplanar image looks much grainier (salt-and-pepper appearance). At the lowest mA settings (**Panel D**), it becomes impossible to rule out significant stenoses and plaques in the mid-segment of this vessel. This situation illustrates the importance of adjusting the tube current to the size of each patient. It is important to note that these images represent simulations, and the differences would be even larger in actual repeated scanning (which would be unethical)

Contrast agent amount [ml] = (10 s + scan duration in sec) × contrast agent flow in ml/s[a]

1st example: 75 kg patient undergoing a 10-s coronary helical scan

(10 s + 10 s) × 4 ml s^{-1} = 80 ml

2nd example: 110 kg patient undergoing a 15-s coronary bypass scan

(10 s + 15 s) × 5 ml s^{-1} = 125 ml

[a] See **Table 7.2** for calculating contrast agent injection rates. The 10 s is a constant.

Table 7.2 Contrast agent injection rates

Body weight	Rate (ml/s)[a]
<60 kg (<132 lb)	3.5
60–80 kg (132–176 lb)	4.0
>80 kg (>176 lb)	5.0

[a] The amount of iodine injected should be about 1.3–2.0 g s^{-1} to ensure adequate opacification of the coronary arteries. The flow rates given in the table are thus valid for contrast agents with an iodine concentration of 350–400 mg ml^{-1}. For contrast agents with a lower iodine concentration (e.g., 320), the flow needs to be increased to achieve the same iodine influx of 1.3–2.0 g s^{-1}. Higher flow rates can also be used with 350–400 mg ml^{-1} contrast agents to make the bolus more compact and increase vessel lumen density (e.g., for stent assessment), but this will also increase the risk of adverse reactions. We feel that the suggestions above are a reasonable compromise between image quality and patient safety

7.1.9 Starting the Scan

Properly connecting the contrast agent line to the patient's intravenous access and making sure that there is no air in the injection system are essential to preventing air from being injected into the cardiac chambers or pulmonary arteries (**Fig. 7.12**). Before starting the contrast agent injection, it is important to reassure the patient that the next breath-hold is the last one and that it takes as long as the one during breath-hold training. Again, mentioning that the patient might feel some warmth can be important for those who are nervous. It is always a good idea to have someone on site to monitor the injection of the contrast agent for at least a few seconds to avoid extravasation.

Immediately prior to injecting the contrast agent, make a "final check" to ensure that the heart rate is still in an acceptable range and the ECG is detected by the system. There are two options for timing the start of the helical scan after intravenous contrast administration: (1) monitoring the arrival of the contrast agent during the injection of the main bolus and starting the helical scan once a threshold has been reached ("bolus tracking"), and (2) injecting a test bolus to determine the individual patient's circulation time and adjust-

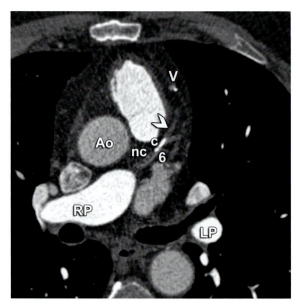

Fig. 7.13 Too-early initiation of the coronary acquisition, with most of the contrast agent still in the pulmonary arteries (LP and RP). As a result, there is very little contrast in the aorta (Ao) and the coronary arteries (*arrowhead*) in this patient with a history of venous coronary bypass grafting (V). Because of the poor opacification, it is very difficult to identify the stenosis in segment 6 of the left anterior descending coronary artery caused by noncalcified (nc) and calcified (c) plaques. In this patient, a test bolus was used to calculate the appropriate delay time for initiation of the coronary scan, but a heart-rate change after contrast agent administration led to incorrect timing of the coronary helical scan. *LP* left pulmonary artery; *RP* right pulmonary artery

ing the scanning parameters accordingly ("test bolus"). The second approach has the disadvantage that any changes between the test bolus and the actual bolus used for coronary opacification (such as relevant heart rate changes) can alter the patient's circulation time. We think that the test bolus approach more commonly leads to mistiming of the coronary helical scan (**Fig. 7.13**), and it has also been shown that the coronary enhancement is less homogenous when this approach is used. We therefore strongly recommend the bolus tracking approach (for 64-slice CT), which also reduces the total amount of contrast agent injected, as no test bolus is needed.

We perform bolus tracking (which should be initiated 10–15 s after the start of contrast injection) by analyzing Hounsfield unit density in a region of interest in the descending aorta (**Fig. 7.9**). The spiral scan at a threshold of 180 Hounsfield units is then initiated. We use the descending aorta, as opposed to the ascending aorta, for example, for bolus tracking because it is less likely for

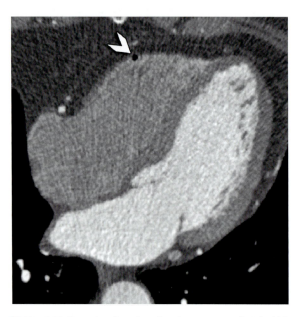

Fig. 7.12 Four-chamber view showing a very small air bubble at the ventral wall of the right ventricle (*arrowhead*). The bubble was most likely introduced when the contrast agent line was connected to the patient's intravenous line. Such small amounts are unlikely to harm the patient. Care must be taken not to inject relevant amounts of air into the cardiac chambers or pulmonary arteries, by properly connecting the contrast agent line and excluding any air that is in the injection system

early-enhancing vessels such as the superior vena cava to affect the region of interest. As soon as the threshold for initiation of the spiral scan has been reached, a simple 5-s breathing instruction is given ("Please breathe in and then hold your breath"). Since there is often a brief increase in heart rate after inspiration, there is an additional gap of 3 s before the helical scan (lasting 8–12 s) is started, so that the heart rate can normalize after submaximal inspiration.

7.1.10 After the Scan

As soon as the prospectively or retrospectively gated coronary scan is completed, we return to the scanning room to make sure that the patient has tolerated the contrast agent well. Because of the nitroglycerin and possible beta blockade, it is advisable that the patient gets up slowly to avoid orthostatic reactions. Most patients are eager to know the results of the examination immediately, which is difficult because a single coronary CT angiography can produce as many as 4,000–5,000 images.

The patient can be offered the opportunity to wait in the seating area after the scan is completed and to meet with the interpreting physician to discuss the results as soon as he or she has finished reading and interpreting the images. This offer is highly appreciated by some patients and many of our referring physicians. In addition, sending reconstructions of the coronary arteries to the referring physician together with the report not only improves further management of the patient but is also a strong marketing tool.

7.2 Reconstruction

Since coronary CT angiography with up to 64 simultaneous detector rows is generally best performed using retrospective ECG gating, image reconstruction is an integral component of the examination. The parameters for coronary and lung reconstructions are compiled in **Table 7.3**, and typical results of these reconstructions are shown in **Fig. 7.14**. The reconstruction of coronary CT angiography is summarized in **List 7.2**.

Table 7.3 Reconstruction settings

	FOV (mm)	Slice thickness (mm)	Reconstruction increment (mm)	Kernel	RR intervals
Coronary images	180–200	0.5–0.75	0.3–0.5	Coronary, possibly stent kernel	0–90% at 10% increments[a] and/or minimal cardiac motion phases
Lung and mediastinal images	Scan field of view[b]	3–5	3–5	Lung and mediastinum	80%[c]

[a] Alternatively, one can reconstruct images at 5% increments around 70–80% of the RR interval

[b] Adapted to included the entire chest in the *xy*-plane

[c] This percentage refers to the center of the reconstruction window (as on Toshiba, Philips, and General Electric scanners). On other scanners (Siemens), the percentage phase given denotes the beginning of the reconstruction phase (which would be equal to approximately 65 or 70% instead)

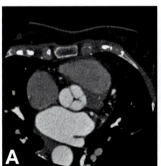 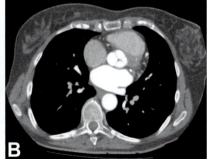 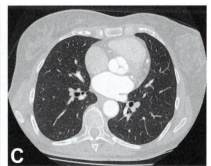

Fig. 7.14 Typical axial images of coronary (**Panel A**), mediastinal (**Panel B**, soft tissue), and lung reconstructions (**Panel C**) at the level of the aortic valve. Please note that the coronary reconstructions here (**Panel A**) were performed on smaller fields of view in order to maximize spatial resolution. The mediastinal (**Panel B**) and lung (**Panel C**) reconstructions are less noisy because of the greater slice thickness (3–5 mm)

> **List 7.2. Steps in the reconstruction of coronary CT images**
>
> 1. Check whether the heart rate was regular throughout scanning
> 2. Perform ECG editing if necessary – consider automatic identification of minimal cardiac motion phases
> 3. Reconstruct coronary axial slices using specific kernels on small fields of view (180–200 mm) – consider stent kernels
> 4. Reconstruct lung and mediastinal axial slices using specific kernels on large fields of view to cover the entire chest width
> 5. Archive all reconstructed coronary images or only those indicated by the reading physician
> 6. Archive all lung and mediastinal images

7.2.1 Slice Thickness and Fields of View

For analysis of the small and tortuous coronary arteries, it is of utmost importance to keep the reconstructed slice thickness for the coronary axial slices as thin as possible. A slice thickness of 3 or 2 mm is clearly inadequate for coronary imaging, but there is also a remarkable difference between 0.5 and 1.0-mm reconstructions (**Fig. 7.15**). The reconstructed slice thickness is different from the reconstruction increment. This increment between the centers of adjacent slices can be thinner (e.g., 0.4 mm) than the slice thickness (e.g., 0.5 mm) to improve the 3D reconstructions by spatial interpolation. However, the true spatial resolution is defined by the actual slice thickness, and a reduction in the slice increment may impose too large a burden on the local picture archiving and communication system. Thus, it clearly depends on the local situation whether it is advisable to use this spatial interpolation approach or not.

What is much more important than slice interpolation is the use of a minimally small reconstruction field of view (ca. 180–200 mm) to make optimal use of the maximal spatial resolution of the scanner (10 line pairs per cm) using a 512 × 512 image matrix (**Table 7.3**). With this image matrix, a 180-mm field of view results in a pixel size of 0.35×0.35 mm^2 (0.12 mm^2). If one inadvertently uses a 320-mm field of view for reconstruction, the resulting pixel size is about 0.625×0.625 mm^2 (0.4 mm^2), which is almost four times larger. The effect on image quality is significant and is illustrated in **Figs. 7.16** and **7.17**. In contrast to the situation for coronary axial slices, it is ethically desirable to use the entire scanned field for reconstruction of the lung, the mediastinum, and the chest wall (**Fig. 7.14** and **Table 7.3**) to avoid overlooking any pathology in this area.

7.2.2 Temporal Resolution and the Cardiac Reconstruction Phase

Temporal resolution is still the major limitation of coronary CT and the main cause of nondiagnostic images, and therefore all possible measures must be taken to improve this parameter. One such measure is adaptive multisegment reconstruction, which should be used whenever available for patients with heart rates greater than 50–60 beats per min (**Figs. 7.18** and **7.19**). An alternative approach that markedly improves temporal resolution is dual-source CT (DSCT), which allows a 50% reduction in the length of the reconstruction window, regardless of the heart rate (**Fig. 7.20**). In this way, DSCT markedly reduces heart-rate dependence, although adaptive multisegment reconstruction is not available on DSCT scanners.

Reconstruction can be done throughout the cardiac cycle at 10% intervals, resulting in 10 phases, or around a mid-diastolic interval at 5% increments (about 70–80% of the RR interval) (**Table 7.3**). Most of the suitable reconstruction phases (intervals) within the cardiac cycles are mid-diastolic phases and end-systolic phases. The latter are especially suitable for analysis in patients with higher heart rates. Reconstruction of several phases throughout the RR interval has the advantage that the resulting data can be used for high-resolution analysis of regional and global cardiac function without having to perform any additional reconstructions. It is important to note that the designations of the phases are not defined consistently by the different vendors. The percentage of the RR interval refers either to the center of the reconstruction phase

Fig. 7.15 Importance of slice collimation for image quality, as shown in curved multiplanar reformations along the right coronary artery (*first column*), left anterior descending coronary artery (*middle column*), and left circumflex coronary artery (*third column*). Slice thicknesses of 3 mm (**Panels A–C**) and 2 mm (**Panels D–F**) are clearly inadequate for coronary imaging, as can be seen in the step-like appearance of the vessel on curved multiplanar reformations. These slice thicknesses were commonly used with electron-beam CT and 4-slice CT. But there is also an image-quality difference (step-like appearance) between 0.5 and 1.0-mm slice thickness reconstructions available on different 16 and 64-slice CT scanners (**Panels G-I** and **Panels J-L**). All reconstructions were performed using raw data that were acquired with 64 by 0.5-mm detector collimation in a single patient

7.2 · Reconstruction

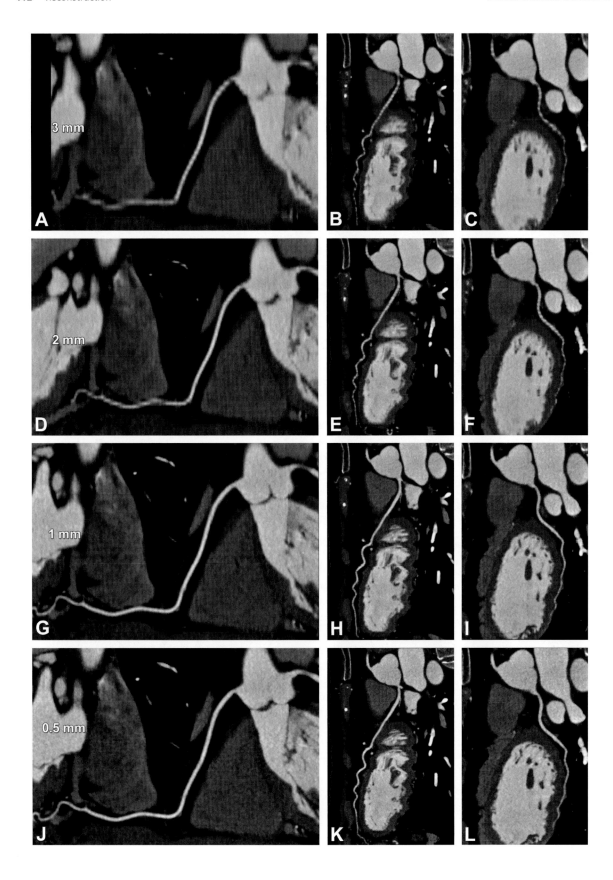

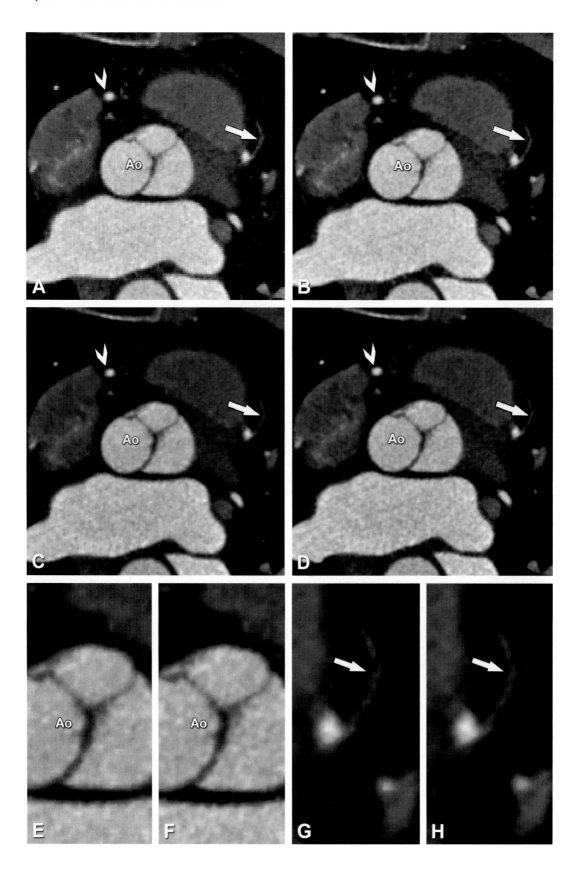

7.2 · Reconstruction

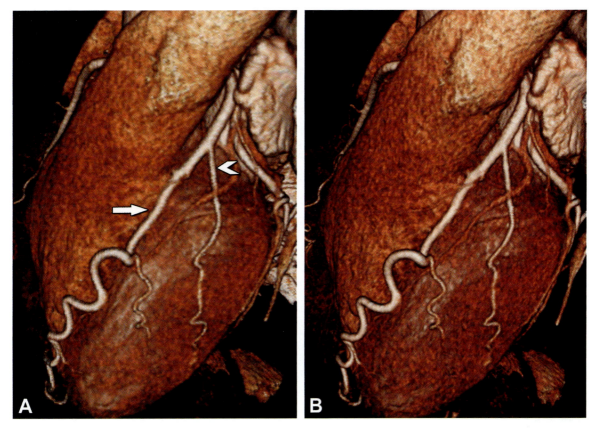

Fig. 7.17 Effect of the reconstruction field of view (320 vs. 180 mm) on the image quality of coronary artery reconstructions. Three-dimensional reconstructions of the LAD (of the same patient as in Fig. 7.16) show the relevantly lower spatial resolution obtained using the 320-mm reconstruction field of view (**Panel A**), when compared with the smaller 180-mm reconstruction field of view (**Panel B**), as illustrated by the mid-LAD (*arrow*) and the first diagonal branch (*arrowhead*)

(Toshiba, Philips, and General Electric) or the beginning of the reconstruction phase (Siemens). As a result, there are different recommendations regarding minimal cardiac motion phases, but these can be matched (thus, the start of the reconstruction phase at about 65–70% of the RR interval corresponds to a center of the phase at about 75–80%). In patients with severe arrhythmias (e.g., atrial fibrillation) an absolute temporal reconstruction approach (in ms) might be superior to relative reconstruction intervals (% of the RR interval).

In discussing the number of phases to be reconstructed and the distance between phases, one must bear in mind that the reconstruction window in coronary CT angiography is about 50–200 ms long, corresponding to about 8–20% of the RR interval. Therefore, there will not be a relevant difference between reconstructions at intervals ≤5%.

Heart rate is crucial in determining the position of the minimal cardiac motion phase that is most suitable for reconstruction. In patients with higher heart rates, end-systolic phases (e.g., 30–40%) are often superior to

Fig. 7.16 Effect of the reconstruction field of view (320 vs. 180 mm) on the image quality of coronary artery reconstructions. The original axial images of the 320-mm reconstruction field of view (**Panel A**) are compared with the 180-mm reconstruction fields of view (**Panel B**). The 320-mm reconstructions (**Panel A**) have markedly poorer spatial resolution with coarser pixels (ca. 0.625 × 0.625 mm² vs. 0.35 × 0.35 mm²), as illustrated by the right coronary artery (*arrowhead*) and a rather small side branch of the LAD (*arrow*). On workstations this difference appears to be somewhat blurred but is still present, as can be seen in the images at exactly the same anatomic level (panel **C** vs. **D**). Magnified views of the aortic valve cusps (**Panel E** vs. **F**) and the small side branch of the LAD (**Panel G** vs. **H**) clearly show the considerable advantage of using small 180-mm reconstruction fields of view (**Panels F** and **H**). *Ao* aorta

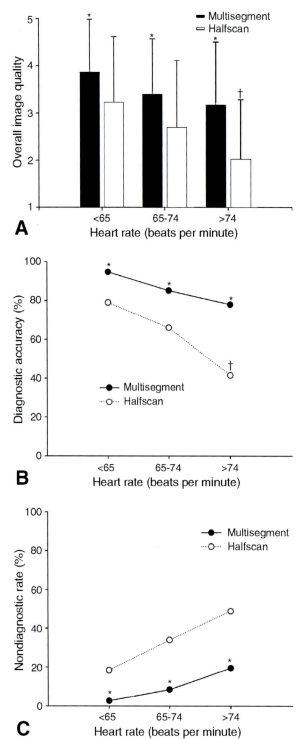

Fig. 7.18 Comparison of overall image quality (**Panel A**), per-patient diagnostic accuracy (**Panel B**), and per-patient nondiagnostic rate (**Panel C**) of CT coronary angiography obtained using adaptive multisegment and standard halfscan reconstructions in three heart rate groups. There is a trend toward reduced overall image quality and accuracy at higher heart rates, which was significant in the case of the halfscan reconstructions when the 65–74 and above 74 beats-per-min groups were compared (*dagger*). Nevertheless, regardless of whether multisegment reconstruction is available or not, the heart rate should be reduced to below 65 beats per min by beta blocker administration whenever possible. For all three heart rate groups, overall image quality, diagnostic accuracy, and nondiagnostic rate are significantly superior for multisegment reconstruction than for standard halfscan reconstruction (*asterisk*). Therefore, whenever available, adaptive multisegment reconstruction should be used instead of halfscan reconstruction. A very recent important alternative to improve temporal resolution is DSCT (**Fig. 7.20**). Note that the image quality and accuracy obtained with multisegment reconstruction at high heart rates (>74 beats per min) are comparable with the results obtained using standard halfscan reconstruction at low heart rates (<65 beats per min). From Dewey et al., Eur Radiol 2007

7.2 • Reconstruction

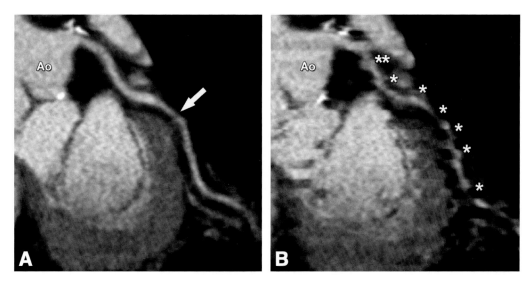

Fig. 7.19 Advantages of multisegment reconstruction (**Panel A**) over halfscan reconstruction (panel **B**), as illustrated by a curved multiplanar reformation along the left circumflex coronary artery (*arrow* depicts stenosis) in a patient with a heart rate of 85–87 beats per min during scanning. There are multiple motion artifacts resulting from insufficient temporal resolution with halfscan reconstruction (*asterisks*), which obscure the stenosis (**Panel B**). Ao aorta

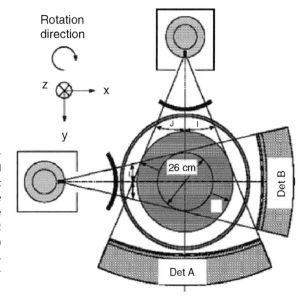

Fig. 7.20 Technical realization of dual-source computed tomography (DSCT). One detector (Det A) covers the entire scan field of view with a diameter of 50 cm, while the other detector (Det B) is restricted to a smaller (25 cm), central field of view because of space limitations on the gantry. In this way, the length of the image reconstruction window can be reduced by a factor of 2 when compared with standard halfscan reconstruction using a single X-ray source, to one-fourth of the gantry rotation time. Thus, temporal resolution is significantly improved. Used with permission from Flohr et al., Eur Radiol 2006

diastolic phases in terms of image quality. Selection of the reconstruction phase has considerable influence on the diagnostic accuracy of coronary CT angiography. It has been shown, for example, that a single reconstruction phase (typically with the center of the reconstruction window at 80%) results in optimal quality and diagnostic accuracy in only half of the patients. Two reconstruction phases are necessary in 40% of patients, and at least three phases in 10%, to optimally evaluate the entire coronary artery tree by CT angiography. Automatic determination of minimal cardiac motion using software approaches based on the raw data (e.g., "Best Phase") using motion

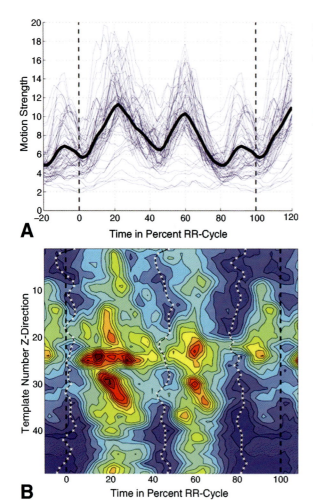

Fig. 7.21 Motion strength curve and motion map samples. **Panel A** shows a representative mean curve of the motion strength function for all voxels within a single axial plane. Motion strength (corresponding to inverse similarity) is plotted against phase point propagation of one cardiac cycle. The *curve* shows low motion troughs for the end-systolic phase (~46%) and the mid-diastolic or diastasis phase (~80%). **Panel B** shows the corresponding motion map, with color-coded (*blue*, low motion; *red*, high motion) motion strength curves plotted against the cardiac phase (*x*-axis) and against *z*-axis propagation of the helical scan (*y*-axis truncated at a value of 50 to confine the coverage to aortic root position, *y*-axis value = 0, down to the diaphragmatic surface of the heart, *y*-axis value = 49). A low-motion phase becomes apparent as a *blue valley* between *red-colored* systolic contraction (0–40% longitudinally) and rapid diastolic filling (50–70% longitudinally). Atrial contraction is apparent as a hump around 90%. *Lines with crosses* track the valleys of lowest motion; *dashed vertical lines* mark the beginning and the end of the cardiac cycle (R to R peak). Used with permission from M. Hoffmann et al., Eur Radiol 2006

maps (**Fig. 7.21**) is likely to considerably simplify identification of the optimal cardiac phase for coronary artery analysis (Chap. 9).

Recommended Reading

1. Achenbach S. Computed tomography coronary angiography. J Am Coll Cardiol 2006; 48:1919–28
2. Cademartiri F, Luccichenti G, Marano R, Runza G, Midiri M. Use of saline chaser in the intravenous administration of contrast material in non-invasive coronary angiography with 16-row multislice Computed Tomography. Radiol Med (Torino) 2004; 107:497–505
3. Cademartiri F, Maffei E, Palumbo AA, et al. Influence of intra-coronary enhancement on diagnostic accuracy with 64-slice CT coronary angiography. Eur Radiol 2008; 18:576–83
4. Cademartiri F, Mollet NR, Runza G, et al. Improving diagnostic accuracy of MDCT coronary angiography in patients with mild heart rhythm irregularities using ECG editing. AJR Am J Roentgenol 2006; 186:634–8
5. Cademartiri F, Mollet NR, Runza G, et al. Influence of intracoronary attenuation on coronary plaque measurements using multislice computed tomography: observations in an ex vivo model of coronary computed tomography angiography. Eur Radiol 2005; 15:1426–31
6. Cademartiri F, Nieman K, van der Lugt A, et al. Intravenous contrast material administration at 16-detector row helical CT coronary angiography: test bolus versus bolus-tracking technique. Radiology 2004; 233:817–23
7. Cademartiri F, Runza G, Mollet NR, et al. Impact of intravascular enhancement, heart rate, and calcium score on diagnostic accuracy in multislice computed tomography coronary angiography. Radiol Med (Torino) 2005; 110:42–51
8. Dewey M, Hamm B. CT Coronary angiography: examination technique, clinical results, and outlook on future developments. Fortschr Röntgenstr 2007; 179:246–60
9. Dewey M, Hoffmann H, Hamm B. Multislice CT coronary angiography: effect of sublingual nitroglycerine on the diameter of coronary arteries. Fortschr Röntgenstr 2006; 178:600–04
10. Dewey M, Laule M, Krug L, et al. Multisegment and halfscan reconstruction of 16-slice computed tomography for detection of coronary artery stenoses. Invest Radiol 2004; 39:223–9
11. Dewey M, Teige F, Laule M, Hamm B. Influence of heart rate on diagnostic accuracy and image quality of 16-slice CT coronary angiography: comparison of multisegment and halfscan reconstruction approaches. Eur Radiol 2007; 17:2829–37
12. Dewey M, Teige F, Rutsch W, Schink T, Hamm B. CT coronary angiography: influence of different cardiac reconstruction intervals on image quality and diagnostic accuracy. Eur J Radiol 2007
13. Einstein AJ, Moser KW, Thompson RC, Cerqueira MD, Henzlova MJ. Radiation dose to patients from cardiac diagnostic imaging. Circulation 2007; 116:1290–305
14. Engelken F, Dewey M. Breathhold trial prior to multislice CT coronary angiography to determine optimal scanning parameters. European Congress of Radiology (ECR) 2008; C-877

15. Flohr TG, McCollough CH, Bruder H, et al. First performance evaluation of a dual-source CT (DSCT) system. Eur Radiol 2006; 16:256–68
16. Hoffmann MH, Lessick J, Manzke R, et al. Automatic determination of minimal cardiac motion phases for computed tomography imaging: initial experience. Eur Radiol 2006; 16:365–73
17. Horiguchi J, Fujioka C, Kiguchi M, et al. Soft and intermediate plaques in coronary arteries: how accurately can we measure CT attenuation using 64-MDCT? AJR Am J Roentgenol 2007; 189:981–8
18. Horiguchi J, Shen Y, Hirai N, et al. Timing on 16-slice scanner and implications for 64-slice cardiac CT: do you start scanning immediately after breath hold? Acad Radiol 2006; 13:173–6
19. Hur G, Hong SW, Kim SY, et al. Uniform image quality achieved by tube current modulation using SD of attenuation in coronary CT angiography. AJR Am J Roentgenol 2007; 189:188–96
20. Husmann L, Valenta I, Gaemperli O, et al. Feasibility of low-dose coronary CT angiography: first experience with prospective ECG-gating. Eur Heart J 2008; 29:191–7
21. Kim DJ, Kim TH, Kim SJ, et al. Saline flush effect for enhancement of aorta and coronary arteries at multidetector CT coronary angiography. Radiology 2008; 246:110–5
22. Leber AW, Johnson T, Becker A, et al. Diagnostic accuracy of dual-source multi-slice CT-coronary angiography in patients with an intermediate pretest likelihood for coronary artery disease. Eur Heart J 2007; 28:2354–60
23. Mahesh M, Cody DD. Physics of cardiac imaging with multiple-row detector CT. Radiographics 2007; 27:1495–509
24. Morin RL, Gerber TC, McCollough CH. Radiation dose in computed tomography of the heart. Circulation 2003; 107: 917–22
25. Paul JF, Abada HT. Strategies for reduction of radiation dose in cardiac multislice CT. Eur Radiol 2007; 17:2028–37
26. Ropers U, Ropers D, Pflederer T, et al. Influence of heart rate on the diagnostic accuracy of dual-source computed tomography coronary angiography. J Am Coll Cardiol 2007; 50:2393–8
27. Schnapauff D, Zimmermann E, Dewey M. Technical and clinical aspects of coronary computed tomography angiography. Semin Ultrasound CT MR 2008; 29:167–75
28. Shapiro MD, Pena AJ, Nichols JH, et al. Efficacy of pre-scan beta-blockade and impact of heart rate on image quality in patients undergoing coronary multidetector computed tomography angiography. Eur J Radiol 2007
29. Yoshimura N, Sabir A, Kubo T, Lin PJ, Clouse ME, Hatahu H. Correlation between image noise and body weight in coronary CTA with 16-row MDCT. Acad Radiol 2006; 13:324–8

Toshiba Aquilion 64

E. Zimmermann

8a.1 Examination 67
8a.1.1 Preparation.. 67
8a.1.2 Defining the Scan Range 67
8a.1.3 SureStart.. 67
8a.1.4 Breath-Hold Training
 and Premedication.................................... 70
8a.2 Reconstruction... 72

Abstract

This chapter outlines how the coronary arteries are examined and reconstructed on Toshiba CT scanners.

8a.1 Examination

8a.1.1 Preparation

The patient is positioned on the scanner table in a comfortable supine position with the arms raised above the head and feet-first. To image the heart in the isocenter of the scanner, the patient should be positioned slightly to the right side of the table. It is recommended that the 20 or 18-gauge cannula be checked by means of a physiologic saline flush immediately before scanning to avoid contrast extravasation. Care must be taken to remove all foreign materials that can cause image artifacts (e.g., electrocardiography electrodes/cables and other metal-dense foreign bodies) from the scan field. It is also important to make sure that the ECG electrodes make good contact with the patient's skin and that a good R-wave is displayed on the monitor (**Fig. 8a.1**). Details of patient preparation for coronary CT angiography on all scanner types are presented in Chaps. 6 and 7.

8a.1.2 Defining the Scan Range

A low-dose planning scan (scanogram with 50 mA) is obtained to define the start and end of the spiral scan, identify the widest dimension of the heart, and place the SureStart (**Figs. 8a.2–8a.4**). The start position is placed just above the origins of the coronary arteries, using the left atrial appendage for orientation. The scan ends just below the heart, and can be stopped manually. The Sure Start is placed at the start of the scan, by positioning the active line exactly over the upper boundary of the scan as illustrated in **Fig. 8a.2**. While placing the line, the user should once more verify the correct start position of the spiral scan. The SureStart should not contain the coronary arteries or be placed too high (**Fig. 8a.4**). Careful planning of the scan is essential for achieving an optimal result while minimizing radiation exposure.

8a.1.3 SureStart

Planning the scan delay using the SureStart bolus tracking tool is illustrated in **Fig. 8a.4**. The selected scan plane, just above the origin of the coronary arteries, is chosen to start the scan at the optimal time by monitoring the arrival of the contrast bolus in a region of interest (ROI) placed in the descending aorta (**Fig. 8a.5**). Important landmarks in this plane are the sternum anteriorly and the descending aorta posteriorly. Also seen in this plane are a segment of the pulmonary trunk and a portion of the anterolateral chest wall. The ROI in the descending aorta is used to monitor the increase in Hounsfield units (HU) after initiation of contrast injection.

The scan delay after contrast injection can be determined in one of the two ways: (1) by injection of a test bolus to determine the patient's individual circulation time and optimize the spiral scan parameters accordingly, or (2) by bolus tracking, with automatic triggering of the scan once a predefined Hounsfield threshold has

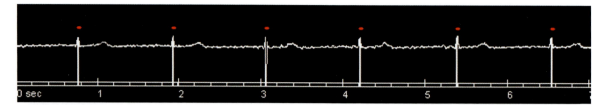

Fig. 8a.1 Illustration of optimal ECG recordings. A clear R-wave and sinus rhythm are essential for reconstruction of the image data. Here, the *red dot* indicates identification of the R-wave. An incorrect R-wave can be removed by clicking on the *red dot* (ECG editing). In patients with arrhythmia, it may be helpful to add "virtual R-waves" by clicking on additional *red dots* or to remove incorrectly identified R-waves. The goal is to obtain a highly regular ECG in order to minimize image artifacts

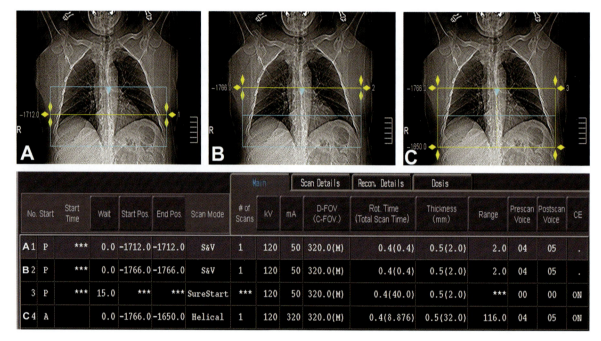

Fig. 8a.2 Planning the acquisition. A planning scan (scanogram) is acquired to identify the greatest circumference of the heart (**Panel A**), position the SureStart (**Panel B**), and define the scan length (**Panel C**) for the subsequent helical coronary examination. *Yellow* indicates the active area, while *blue* indicates inactive areas. As anatomical structures may be displaced as a result of respiratory motion, we recommend defining the start of the scan about 1 cm above the assumed coronary artery origins and the end of the scan about 1 cm below the heart base. **Panel A** shows a single slice (low-dose scan, 50 mA) that defines the greatest circumference of the heart. **Panel B** shows another low-dose single slice (50 mA) (**Fig. 8a.4**) that defines the SureStart, which serves to trigger the spiral scan once the desired density threshold has been reached. The scan is automatically started after 15 s. **Panel C** defines the scan length. The start of the spiral scan corresponds to the SureStart position. The tube current for the spiral scan is selected according to the patient's weight and is higher in obese patients to ensure an adequate image quality

been reached (**Figs. 8a.4** and **8a.5**). Use of the test bolus method increases the total amount of contrast injected and may be inaccurate because the circulation time may vary. Contrast agent injection is usually followed by an automatic 40-ml intravenous saline flush administered at a flow rate of 4 ml s^{-1}, which serves to wash out the right ventricle and improve coronary artery visualization.

Precontrast baseline attenuation is also measured in the descending aorta. In our experience, good results are achieved using a threshold of 180 HU when baseline attenuation is in the range of approximately 30–60 HU. On the basis of our experience, we recommend the use of the SureStart bolus tracking option because it consistently yields good-quality images.

8a.1 · Examination

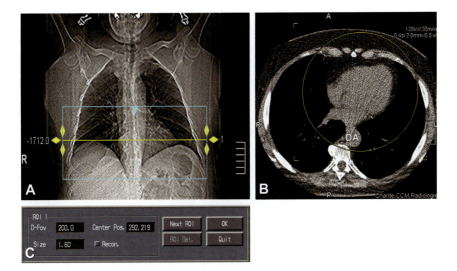

Fig. 8a.3 Defining the FoV. The scan depicting the greatest circumference of the heart (**Panel A**) is used to define the FoV (**Panel B**) according to individual heart size, ensuring good image quality at the highest possible spatial resolution. In the majority of patients, if the FoV should be about 180–200 mm (**Panel C**), the FoV should comprise the descending aorta (DA) and part of the anterior chest wall. The descending aorta is more suitable for measuring contrast inflow than the ascending aorta because it is associated with fewer motion artifacts

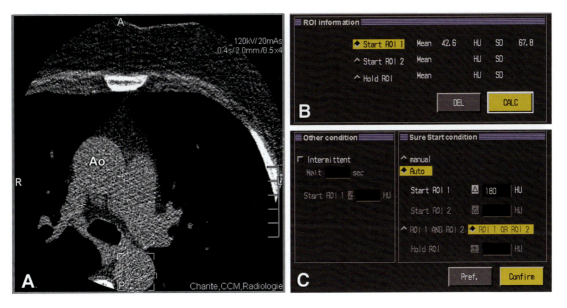

Fig. 8a.4 Planning of the SureStart. Using the SureStart (**Fig. 8a.2**), a ROI is identified in the descending aorta (*circle* in **Panel A**); this region should be neither too large nor too small, in order to avoid mistriggering the spiral scan. The ROI is placed in the descending aorta because there are fewer motion artifacts than in the ascending aorta (Ao). In this way, it is possible to avoid mistriggering of the scan as a result of effects of the superior vena cava, which is opacified very early. Another safeguard is checking attenuation in the ROI (**Panel A**) by clicking on "CALC" (calculation in **Panel B**). An attenuation of about 40 HU is optimal. Next, the threshold of 180 HU for starting the scan is defined (**Panel C**), and "Auto" is selected from the menu as the start position. The scan is then automatically started once the 180 HU threshold has been reached. Alternatively, the scan can be started manually by the examiner, on the basis of visual identification of the time of optimal contrast enhancement. Starting the scan manually results in considerable variation in coronary opacification, since the start is influenced by various factors such as the individual's reaction time and the examiner's level of experience

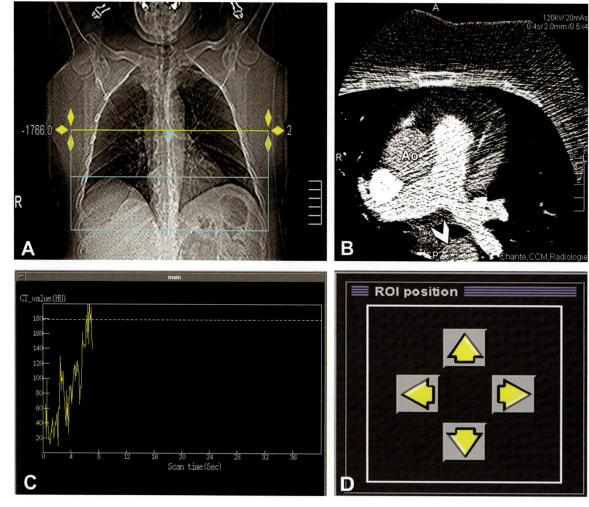

Fig. 8a.5 Start of the helical coronary examination. The position of the SureStart has been defined on the basis of the planning scan (**Panel A**). Next, a continuous low-dose scan (30–50 mA) is acquired at the level of the start of the spiral scan for triggering the spiral scan after IV contrast administration (**Panel B**). Contrast arrival can be tracked in real time. The continuous scan is started not earlier than 15 s after initiation of contrast administration for reasons of radiation protection and to ensure optimal opacification of the target vessels. Contrast arrival is measured in an ROI in the descending aorta (*arrowhead* and *small circle* in **Panel B**). The continuous increase in HU in the ROI over time is represented in **Panel C** in the form of a *graph*. The breathing command starts once the defined threshold of 180 HU has been reached. The scan then starts with a 3-s delay to allow the heart rate to normalize after inspiration. The *arrows* in **Panel D** represent cursor movements and can be clicked to correct the position of the ROI in the descending aorta if necessary. *Ao* ascending aorta

8a.1.4 Breath-Hold Training and Premedication

We recommend sublingual nitroglycerin administration (0.8–1.2 mg) before the breath-hold training. Nitroglycerin dilates the coronary arteries and improves the comparability of the CT findings with those of cardiac catheterization. The effect of nitroglycerin lasts for about 10–30 min. Although nitroglycerin is usually well tolerated, patients should be monitored for the occurrence of possible hemodynamic side effects (e.g., hypotension).

In our department, we use an automatic speech system for the breathing commands ("Please breathe in and hold your breath"). The required breath-hold period is about 6–30 s, depending on the scanner used and the scan volume. Breath-hold training is done without radiation exposure, and the physician or technician should stand next to the patient to verify that the patient can hold his/her breath in submaximal inspiration for the required period and also to check for possible ECG alterations during inspiration. Toshiba scanners have a

8a.1 · Examination

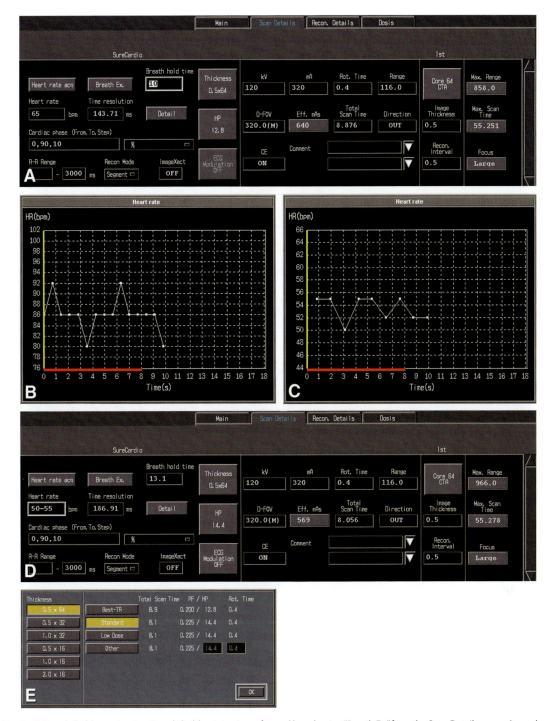

Fig. 8a.6 Breath-hold examination. Breath-hold training is performed by selecting "Breath Ex." from the Scan Details menu. As can be seen in **Panel A**, the default breath-hold time should be 10 s for scanning of the coronary arteries. When bypasses are scanned, longer breath-hold periods are needed according to the scan length. The test is started by clicking on "Breath Ex."; the breathing commands that will also be used during the actual scan are then heard. The computer automatically calculates heart rate variability (which should be <10%) and the optimal helical pitch (HP). **Panel B** shows a case in which heart rate variability is in the upper normal range (80–92 beats per min). **Panel C** shows the results of a second test at a later time after intravenous beta blocker administration. The result is good, with a heart rate of 50–55 beats per min, and the examination can proceed. **Panel D** shows the results of the breath-hold test: a breath-hold time of 13.1 s, total scan time of 8.056 s, heart rate of 50–55 beats per min, and a recommended HP of 14.4. Other recommended scan parameters are shown in **Panel E**

special function for breath-hold training. Heart rate variability should be less than 10% to achieve good results (**Fig. 8a.6**). Breath-hold training can be repeated if the ECG is suboptimal. If intravenous beta blocker injection is deemed necessary, it can be done at this stage. Heart rate variability is determined to allow for individual adjustment of scan parameters such as pitch and gantry rotation time. A consistent level of image quality is achieved in all patients if the tube current is adjusted according to body weight (Chap. 7).

8a.2 Reconstruction

Following acquisition of the CT dataset, a few more steps are necessary to ensure good image quality as a basis for a reliable diagnosis. Motion of the individual coronary arteries, and even of their segments, varies during the different phases of the cardiac cycle. A number of reconstruction algorithms are available to depict the entire coronary arteries without motion. A basic prerequisite, as already mentioned, is sinus rhythm and low

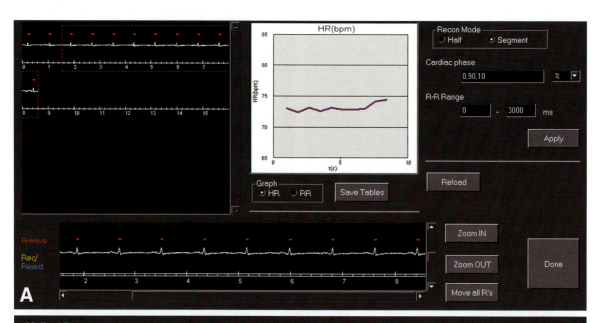

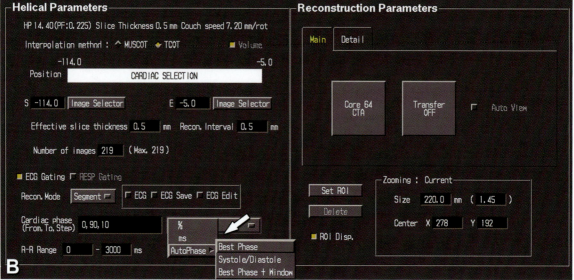

Fig. 8a.7 Caption see opposite page

8a.2 • Reconstruction

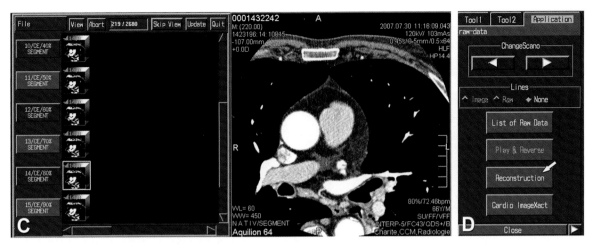

Fig. 8a.7 The reconstruction procedure. **Panel A** shows the ECG and heart rate variability [HR (bmp)] during scanning. The *red dots* indicate the R-waves identified. In **Panel B**, the reconstruction algorithm can be seen. In our example, we use adaptive multisegment reconstruction from 0–90% in increments of 10. These parameters are shown at the bottom of the dialogue window (0, 90, 10). The "Effective slice thickness" is 0.5 mm, and the reconstruction interval ("Recon. Interval") is 0.5 mm. In addition, "BestPhase" and "Systole/Diastole" reconstruction can be selected separately (*arrow*). The effective slice thickness and reconstruction interval are the same. The reconstruction FoV should be 180–220 mm for the coronary arteries and 320 mm for lung/soft tissue reconstruction (**Panel B**, *bottom right*). To send the images to the archive or a workstation, click on the "Transfer off" button to activate the transfer ("Transfer on") and select the target. The reconstructed segment is indicated in **Panel C** (*bottom right*), and any reconstructed image can be selected from a list (**Panel C**, *left part*). Finally, click on "Reconstruction" (*arrow*) to start the reconstruction (**Panel D**)

heart rate variability during data acquisition. Whether this has been the case during scanning should be verified by checking the ECG before proceeding to the next steps (**Fig. 8a.7**).

Image reconstruction starts automatically after completion of the examination, if this option has been selected in the scan protocol. In our department, we use adaptive multisegment reconstruction in increments of 10 from 0–90% (**Fig. 8a.7**). Instead of percent-related or millisecond-related reconstructions, one can opt for so-called "BestPhase" and "Systole/ Diastole" reconstructions. The "BestPhase" always corresponds to either "systole" or "diastole." For "Systole" reconstruction, the systolic phase with the least coronary motion is reconstructed. The same holds true for "Diastole" reconstruction. To reduce storage requirements, one can select "Systole/Diastole" reconstruction alone as the standard option and then, after reviewing the images, retrospectively select individual phases for repeat reconstruction. On the basis of the scan field of view (FoV) selected before the examination, one should then reconstruct the so-called lung and soft tissue windows on large FoVs (**Fig. 8a.8**). It is quite common that accessory pulmonary, soft-tissue, or vascular changes are detected on the noninvasive coronary angiography scans. We use Vitrea workstations for the evaluation of noninvasive coronary angiography and generation of representative images for the patient and referring physician (**Fig. 8a.9**).

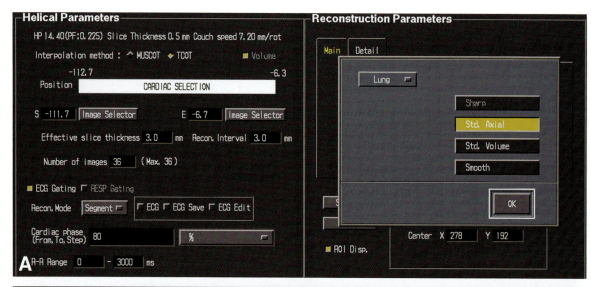
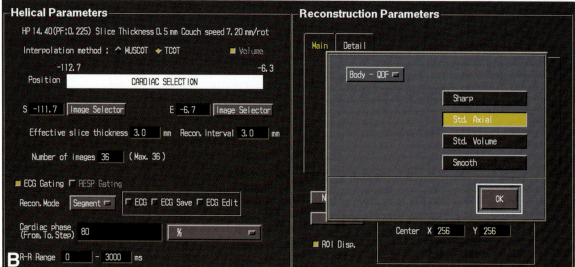

Fig. 8a.8 Reconstruction of lung and soft tissue windows. The lung window (**Panel A**) and soft tissue window (**Panel B**) are reconstructed on large FoVs with an "Effective slice thickness" of 3 mm and a "Recon. Interval" of 3 mm at 80% of the R-R interval and are selected by clicking on "Lung Std. axial" and "Body Std. Axial," respectively. Again, reconstruction is started by clicking on "Reconstruction"

8a.2 • Reconstruction

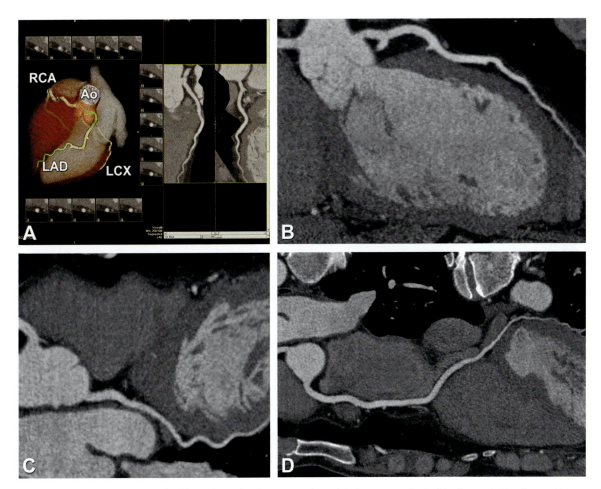

Fig. 8a.9 Reconstruction examples: Three-dimensional reconstructions of the heart are well suited for demonstrating the most important findings. The heart can be rotated to allow viewing from any direction (**Panel A**). An automatic tool identifies a vessel and traces a path along its course for generation of a curved multiplanar reformation (MPR). In this way, the vessel is straightened and displayed in one plane. **Panel B** shows the curved MPR of the left anterior descending coronary artery (LAD). MPR is a fast and easy reconstruction method that provides good image quality and is very helpful in detecting and quantifying coronary stenosis. **Panel C** shows the curved MPR of the left circumflex coronary artery (LCX). **Panel D** shows the MPR of the right coronary artery (RCA). *Ao* ascending aorta

Siemens Somatom Sensation and Definition

C. Klessen

8b.1 Preparing the Examination 77
8b.2 Image Acquisition 77
8b.3 Image Reconstruction 81
8b.4 Dual-Source CT ("Somatom Definition") 84

Abstract

This chapter describes the acquisition and reconstruction of coronary CT angiography data sets on Siemens scanners.

8b.1 Preparing the Examination

The vendor recommends performing coronary angiography with the patient in a supine head-first position. Nevertheless, scanning the patient in feet-first position has some advantages: The patient is easier to monitor and can be accessed more quickly in case of an emergency (e.g., contrast medium intolerance or extravasation). Moreover, it is easier to administer intravenous beta blockers or nitroglycerin spray and other medications. Note, however, that the speakers for giving instructions are at the back of the gantry. Thus, the volume must be turned up when examining patients in the feet-first position, especially if they are hard of hearing.

It is important to place the ECG electrodes outside the scan area to reduce image artifacts. Correct electrode placement is illustrated in **Fig. 8b.1**. Moreover, with the Somatom Sensation 64, which uses a unique z-flying focal spot technology with 32 simultaneous detector rows, the ECG electrodes must be in place before the scan protocol is called up in order for the software to recognize the ECG signal. Details of patient preparation for coronary CT angiography on all scanner types are presented in Chaps. 6 and 7.

8b.2 Image Acquisition

Acquisition of a conventional chest topogram (**Fig. 8b.2**) is followed by planning and acquiring two axial control scans (**Fig. 8b.3**). The first control scan is acquired in the plane with the largest transverse extension of the heart and serves to optimize the field of view for the subsequent CT angiogram (**Fig. 8b.3**). To further reduce radiation exposure, this scan may be skipped; the field of view for the CT angiography scan can alternatively be planned on the real-time images acquired during the scan. Optimal spatial resolution is achieved by selecting a small field of view for image reconstruction. The second control scan is obtained to select the scan position for test bolus acquisition (**Fig. 8b.3**). The subsequent test bolus scan consists of a series of images acquired at rate of one image per second (**Fig. 8b.4**). The test bolus consists of 10–15 ml of iodine-based contrast medium, followed by a 30- to 50-ml saline flush (injection rate: 5 ml s^{-1}) in normal-weight patients. Radiation exposure is minimized by starting the scan 10–15 s after injection and stopping acquisition once the contrast medium peak has been reached. A dedicated software tool, DynEva, is available for automatic analysis of the test bolus series.

Next, the CT angiography scan, which is acquired from top to bottom, is planned (**Fig. 8b.5**). In patients with a constant low heart rate (≤60 beats per min), prospective ECG dose modulation (ECG pulsing) can be used, thereby reducing the radiation exposure by up to 40–50%. In slender patients, radiation exposure can be considerably reduced by using a 100 kV scan protocol. The scan delay (the time interval between the start of the test bolus injection and image acquisition) is the individual test bolus time plus an additional 3 s. The additional 3 s delay time is needed to obtain optimal arterial contrast in the ascending aorta and the coronary arteries on the

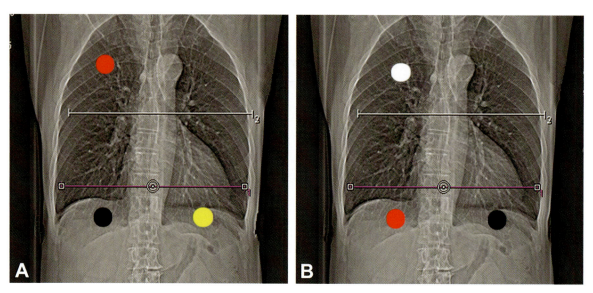

Fig. 8b.1 Optimal positioning of the ECG electrodes on the chest. **Panel A** shows the IEC standard and **Panel B**: the USA standard

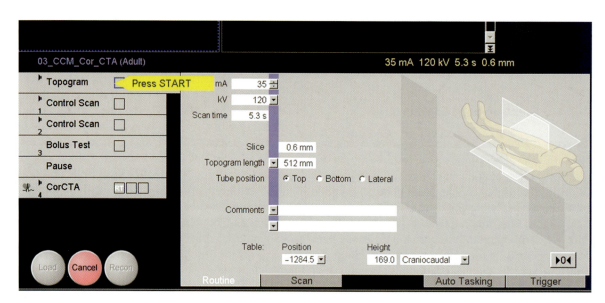

Fig. 8b.2 The first step is the acquisition of a chest topogram (scanogram), typically acquired from top to bottom. To minimize the scan area, the acquisition can be stopped as soon as the entire heart has been scanned

Fig. 8b.4 Bolus test scan. The test scan comprises a maximum of 40 images. It is started 10–15 s after the beginning of the contrast medium injection. The test bolus series can be analyzed visually or with the DynEva software (**Panel B–D**). A region of interest (ROI) is defined in the ascending aorta for analysis (**Panel B**). The time to peak can be read in a table (*arrow* in **Panel C**) after entering the delay used for image acquisition (*arrow* in **Panel D**)

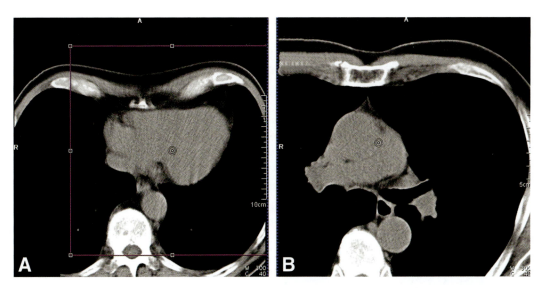

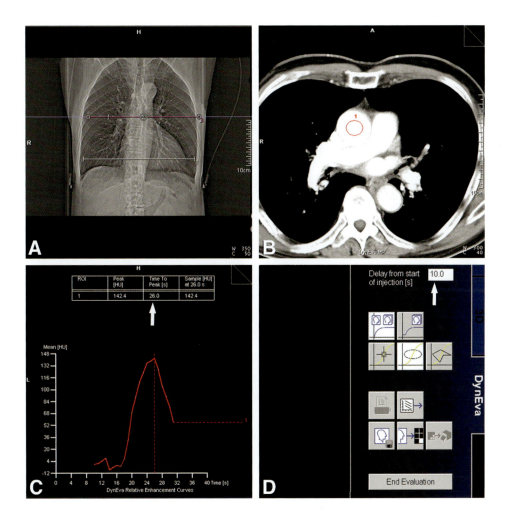

Fig. 8b.3 Acquisition of two control scans. The first control scan (**Panel A**) is positioned at the level of the greatest transverse extension of the cardiac silhouette on the topogram and serves to plan the field of view for the coronary CT angiography scan. The second control scan (**Panel B**) is obtained about 1–2 cm below the tracheal bifurcation to identify the position for test bolus acquisition

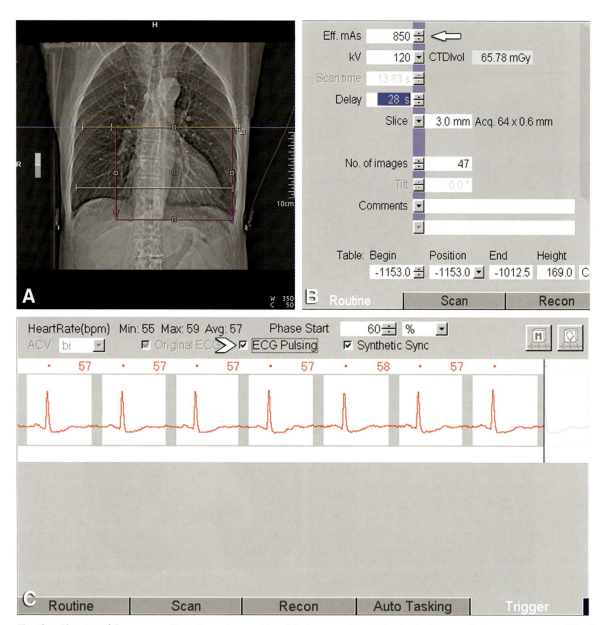

Fig. 8b.5 Planning of the coronary CT angiography scan (**Panel A**). For normal-weight patients, the manufacturer recommends 850 eff. mAs (*arrow* in **Panel B**). In slender patients, radiation exposure can be considerably reduced by using a 100 kV protocol. The highest possible eff. mAs value may be required in obese patients. Finally, prospective ECG dose modulation (ECG pulsing) can be activated from the trigger card of the Syngo menu (*arrowhead* in **Panel C**)

8b.3 Image Reconstruction

one hand and low contrast in the right ventricle and the right atrium on the other, in order to avoid inflow artifacts that may hamper the evaluation of the right coronary artery. To minimize the inferior extension of the scan field, scanning can be manually discontinued as soon as the real-time images show the entire heart.

The first step in image reconstruction is to check the recorded ECG (**Fig. 8b.6**). If there are isolated extrasystoles, the corresponding reconstruction intervals can be deactivated or deleted for image reconstruction. It

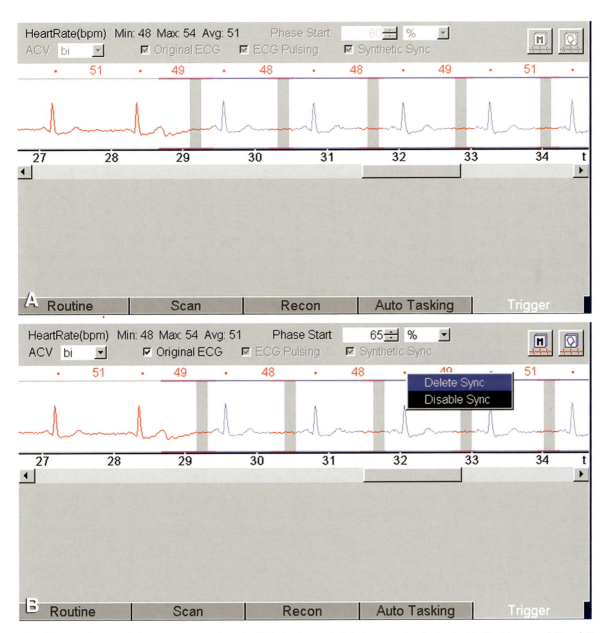

Fig. 8b.6 As a first step in image reconstruction, the ECG signal recorded during scanning is checked in the trigger card (**Panel A**). The minimum, maximum, and average heart rate during the acquisition are displayed on the top of the trigger card. If isolated extrasystoles are present, the corresponding reconstruction intervals can be deactivated or deleted (**Panel B**)

is recommended that a preview series be generated at this point on the basis of a reference image at the level of the mid-RCA (segment 2) to identify the most suitable phase for image reconstruction (**Fig. 8b.7**). Next, thick slices and thin slices are reconstructed at the optimal phase of the RR interval determined in this way (**Fig. 8b.8**). Reconstruction is usually done using a soft-tissue reconstruction algorithm (B25f smooth), while a sharper kernel (B 46f) may be used to improve the evaluation of calcified plaques and stents. Alternatively, multiphasic reconstructions (i.e., automatic reconstruction of multiple phases of the RR interval) can be performed. Multiphasic reconstructions (e.g., 0–90% in 10% intervals) are especially useful if the diagnostic question includes the assessment of ventricular and/or valvular function. In contrast to the situation for the scanners from the other three vendors, the percentage that determines the position of the phase within the RR interval indicates the start, and not the center, of the image reconstruction window (phase). Finally, reconstruction series with a large field of view are computed for assessment of the soft tissue and lungs (**Fig. 8b.9**).

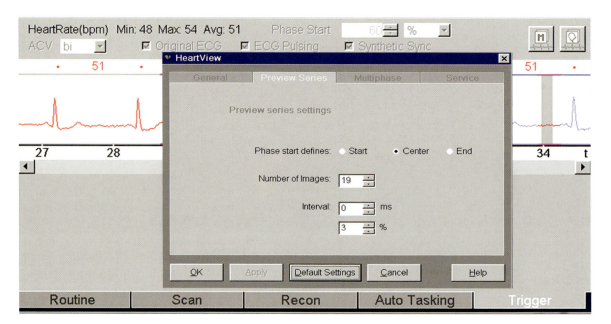

Fig. 8b.7 The user can identify the best time point in the RR interval for image reconstruction by clicking on the "Preview Series" button to generate a series of preliminary images. Such a series may consist for example of 19 images reconstructed at 3% intervals around the start phase. The image selected for generation of the preview series should contain the middle portion of the RCA (segment 2), which is highly susceptible to degradation by motion artifacts

8b.3 • Image Reconstruction

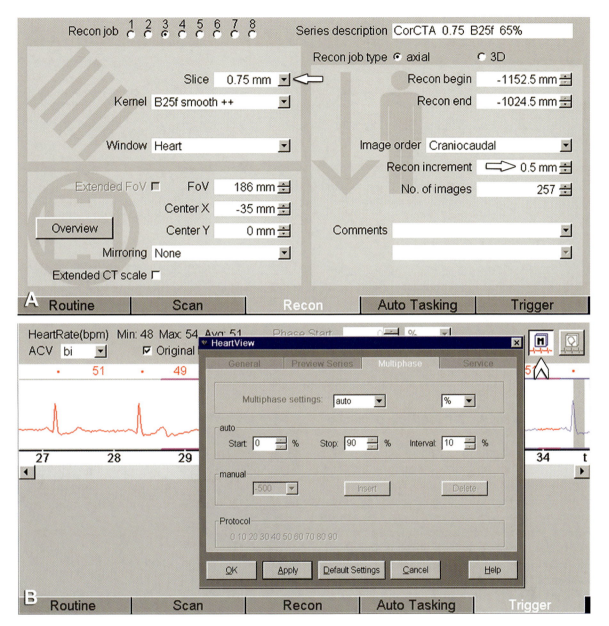

Fig. 8b.8 Next, image series are reconstructed at specific times in the RR interval (**Panels A** and **B**). The time is preselected in the trigger card. As a rule, 0.75 mm images are reconstructed at overlapping intervals (*arrows* in **Panel A**). Alternatively, multiple phases can be automatically reconstructed (in the example shown, from 0–90% of the RR interval at 10% increments). The automatic reconstruction mode is activated by clicking on the multiphase button (*arrowhead* in **Panel B**) and selecting the desired start and stop points as well as the reconstruction interval. Note, however, that the automatic mode generates a large number of images, especially when small intervals are preselected

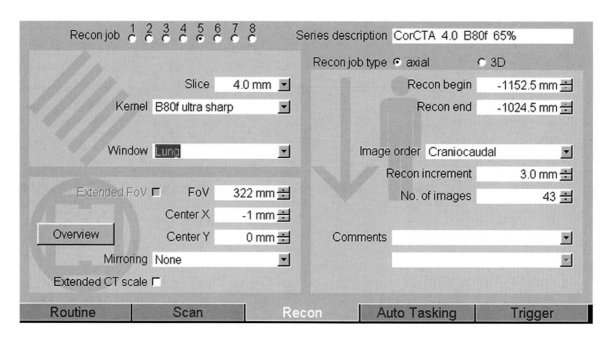

Fig. 8b.9 For evaluation of the lungs, a reconstruction series is generated with a large field of view and thicker slices, using a lung kernel

8b.4 Dual-Source CT ("Somatom Definition")

The technical background of dual-source CT (DSCT) has been described in Chap. 7. The most important practical advantage of DSCT is the improved temporal resolution resulting in better image quality in patients with higher heart rates and arrhythmia (**Fig. 8b.10**). Although beta blockade is recommended to lower heart rates for DSCT as well, the threshold up to which very good image quality can be expected is increased to about 70 beats per min (in contrast to the 60 beats per min threshold with halfscan reconstruction and 64-slice CT). The workflow of scanning using DSCT (Somatom Definition) and the scanner's software is not relevantly different from that of the Somatom Sensation 64. It should be noted that the field of view is limited with dual-source CT because the second gantry has a scan field of only 25 cm. Typical image acquisition parameters are listed in **Table 8b.1**.

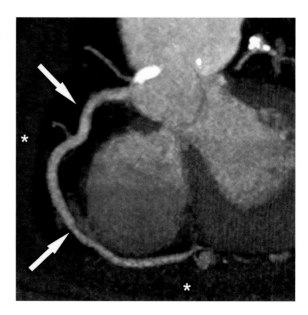

Fig. 8b.10 Example of an examination with dual-source CT in a patient with a heart rate of 125 beats per min. Maximum-intensity projection of the right coronary artery (*arrows*). Note the surrounding pericardial effusion (*asterisks*) that caused the high heart rate. Used with permission from Achenbach et al., Eur Radiol 2008

8b.4 • Dual-Source CT ("Somatom Definition")

Table 8b.1 Typical data acquisition parameters for dual-source CT coronary angiography

Parameter	Value
Gantry rotation time	330 ms
Total scan time	7–10 s
Slice width	0.6 mm
Collimation	19.2 mm
Pitch	0.20 for heart rate <50 beats per min 0.22 for heart rate 50–59 beats per min 0.28 for heart rate 60–69 beats per min 0.33 for heart rate 70–79 beats per min 0.39 for heart rate 80–89 beats per min 0.44 for heart rate 90–99 beats per min 0.50 for heart rate ≥100 beats per min
Tube voltage	120 kV 100 kV for patients <85 kg 80 kV for very slim patients
Tube current	e.g., 400 + 400 mA
mAs value per rotation	e.g., 264 mAs (=800 × 0.33); the resulting value is relevant for image quality considerations
Effective mAs value	e.g., 528 mAs (=267 × 0.6/0.3); in this example, a pitch of 0.3 and an ECG pulsing efficiency factor of 0.6 were assumed; the resulting value is relevant for dose considerations
Contrast agent	50–80 ml at 5 ml s^{-1} (consider 6 ml s^{-1} in patients >100 kg)
Contrast timing	Test bolus or bolus tracking

Modified and used with permission from Achenbach et al., Eur Radiol 2008

Philips Brilliance 64

O. Klass and M. Jeltsch

8c.1	Retrospective Helical Image Acquisition	87
8c.1.1	Scan Protocol	87
8c.2	Prospective Axial Acquisition ("Step & Shoot")	89
8c.2.1	Scan Protocol	89
8c.2.2	Dose Indication Box	91
8c.2.3	Injection Protocol	91
8c.3	Reconstruction	92

Abstract

Performing coronary CT angiography on Philips scanners is described.

8c.1 Retrospective Helical Image Acquisition

After entering the patient's ID, table position, and age group, the desired exam protocol group should be selected (**Fig. 8c.1**). The patient is then placed on the CT table in a supine position, and ECG leads are attached. The automatically started ECG viewer enables permanent registration of heart rate and rhythm including calculation of standard deviation and mean heart rate. Details of patient preparation for coronary CT angiography on all scanner types are presented in Chaps. 6 and 7.

8c.1.1 Scan Protocol

Each examination starts with a surview (scanogram) to determine the position of the heart. The localizer scan should be as small as possible while covering the entire heart and is acquired during a single inspiratory breath-hold.

The scan area for a standard coronary CT angiography is often determined using the tracheal bifurcation as the upper reference point. It is also the level of the plane in which the tracker for the bolus timing algorithm is placed. The scan ends about 1–2 cm below the heart (**Fig. 8c.2**). The scanner gantry isocenter line should be properly placed in the center of the heart. Finally, the entire heart is examined with ECG gating during a single inspiratory breath-hold.

The scan is timed to coincide with peak contrast enhancement, derived from the preceding bolus tracking. Bolus tracking is performed by a Locator and a Tracker scan, positioned on the level of the tracheal bifurcation. Pressing "Go" starts the Locator scan, and the system automatically shows the tracker window. A region of interest (ROI) is positioned in the descending aorta (**Fig. 8c.2**). Now bolus tracking and injection of contrast medium must be started at the same time. After a start delay, several transverse sections are successively acquired at the defined level. The scan starts automatically once attenuation enhancement values in Hounsfield units reach a predefined threshold.

In most patients, helical retrospective gating is used for data acquisition. A standardized examination protocol (**Table 8c.1**) with 64 by 0.625 mm collimation, pitch of 0.2 and a tube rotation time of 400 ms is used. The typical tube voltage is 120 kV with a tube current of 600–900 mAs, depending on patient size, body mass index, and thoracic diameters in the scan area. A standard patient with 75 kg body weight is scanned with 120 kV and a tube voltage of 800 mAs. A separate dose indication box gives the expected dose exposure and scan time (**Fig. 8c.2**).

After the scan is completed, preview images are presented to validate all the required data. Philips also offers an option for editing of the ECG wave as well as off-line arrhythmia handling prior to the start of reconstruction (**Fig. 8c.3**).

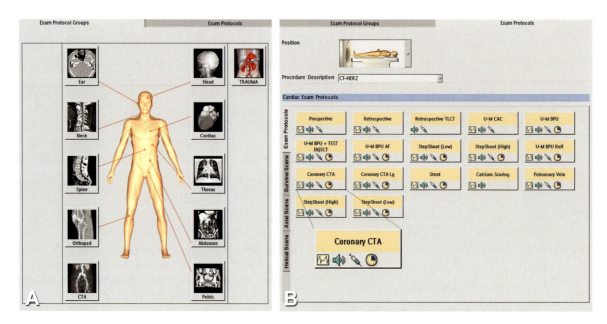

Fig. 8c.1 Setting up the scan protocol. The different "Exam Protocol Groups" are shown in **Panel A** while **Panel B** details the "Cardiac Exam Protocols" such as "Coronary CTA". Depending on the planned examination, you can select between different protocols (e.g., standard helical "Coronary CTA," "Step & Shoot" mode, or "Calcium Scoring")

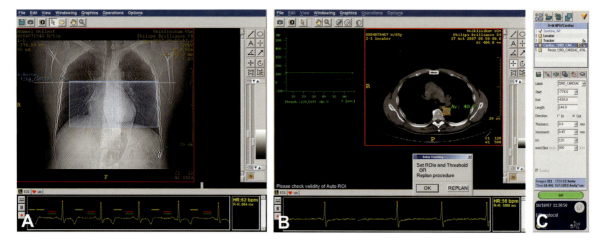

Fig. 8c.2 The user interface for a standard retrospective helical scan, including the defined field of view and an ECG viewer, is shown in **Panel A**. The *blue box* indicates the preselected scan area and range. For bolus tracking, the ROI is positioned in the descending aorta (**Panel B**). The dose indication box shows the expected dose exposure and scan time (**Panel C**)

8c.2 Prospective Axial Acquisition ("Step & Shoot")

Table 8c.1 Typical scan parameters

	Helical scan	Step & Shoot
Total collimation	64 × 0.625 mm	64 × 0.625 mm
Rotation time	400 ms	400 ms
Tube voltage	120–140 kV	
Current time product/tube load	600–900 mAs[a]	150–210 mAs[a]
Pitch	0.2	NA
$CTDI_{vol}$	34–75 mGy[b]	11–22 mGy
Maximum field of view	500 mm	250 mm
Scan duration	Approximately 10 s	Approximately 10 s
ECG synchronization	Retrospective ECG gating	Prospective ECG gating (triggering)
Cycles	NA	4–5
Threshold for bolus tracking	150 HU	150 HU
Postthreshold delay	5–7 s	7 s

NA not applicable
[a] True mAs = electrical mAs; effective mAs = electrical mAs divided by pitch
[b] Without temporal dose modulation ("ECG gating")

For patients with a stable heart rate below 65 beats per min, Philips offers a prospective scan protocol called "Step & Shoot." This new scan type combines the advantages of axial and helical scans and relies on sequential axial acquisitions. Generally, "Step & Shoot" involves a typical scan sequence that is based on volume acquisition ("Shoot") and table movement ("Step"). The heart is covered in four to six axial rotations, combined with prospective triggering (**Fig. 8c.4**). The main advantages of "Step & Shoot" scanning are summarized in **List 8c.1**.

8c.2.1 Scan Protocol

A standardized protocol is also used for prospective acquisition (**Table 8c.1**), with 64 by 0.625 mm collimation and a tube rotation time of 400 ms. The tube voltage is 120–140 kV, and tube current typically 210 mAs. Data are acquired for a full rotation (360°) instead of a half scan plus fan angle to allow for more flexibility in compensating for changes in heart rate.

The planning on the scanogram of the "Step & Shoot" scan is similar to the helical scan with the following differences: The field of view is limited to 250 mm (in both standard and detailed resolutions). This limitation is indicated by a "gray box" that is displayed on the surview image (**Fig. 8c.7**). To make sure that the optimal phase is acquired even under changing conditions, the "Step & Shoot" application has a built-in mechanism that analyzes the patient's heart rate online during the scan, and, if arrhythmia occurs, it responds accordingly. The new reconstruction capabilities of "Step & Shoot" allow the user to select any reconstructed slice thickness and slice increment as in equivalent helical

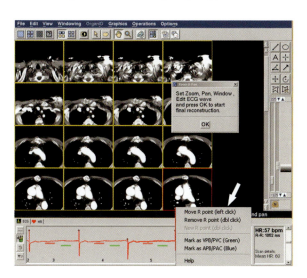

Fig. 8c.3 Preview images shown after completion of scan acquisition. Images can be centered and zoomed to the optimal size. Prior to starting final image reconstruction the ECG of the acquired scan can be manipulated using the off-line arrhythmia handling software as shown in the pop-up window (*arrow*)

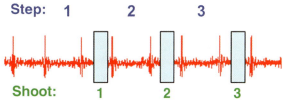

Fig. 8c.4 The principle of sequential axial acquisition after table movement (Step), combined with prospective ECG gating (triggering)

List 8c.1. Advantages and disadvantages of prospective coronary acquisition

Advantages:

1. Provides a low-dose scan: a dose reduction to one-fourth that of standard helical scans
2. Allows each volume to be reconstructed from a single cardiac cycle
3. Includes an online arrhythmia handling mechanism (**Fig. 8c.5**)

Disadvantages:

1. Limited to patients with stable heart rates below 65 beats per min
2. Lower temporal resolution when compared with helical scans
3. Geometric distortion at the borders of the prospectively acquired slabs (**Fig. 8c.6**)

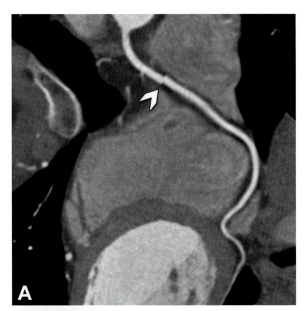

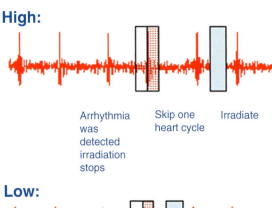

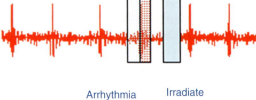

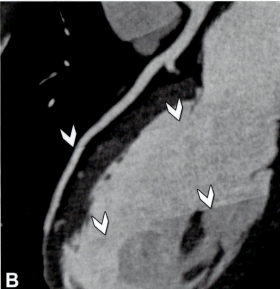

■ **Fig. 8c.5** Two options are available for online arrhythmia handling in the "Step & Shoot" mode. "High" arrhythmia tolerance: When an arrhythmia is detected, irradiation stops immediately; the system waits for one cardiac cycle and then continues exposure in the same table position after the next cycle. "Low" arrhythmia tolerance: When an arrhythmia is detected, irradiation stops immediately; the system continues exposure in the same table position in the cycle immediately following. To prevent excessively long scan times (in the "High" tolerance mode), in a sequence of more than two irregularities, the "High" strategy is automatically changed to "Low"

■ **Fig. 8c.6** Drawbacks of the "Step & Shoot" approach. Curved multiplanar reformations of the right coronary artery with "steps" (*arrowhead* in **Panel A**) and of the left anterior descending coronary artery showing "bands" (*arrowheads* in **Panel B**) as artifacts resulting from geometric distortion at borders of the prospectively acquired slabs

8c.2 • Prospective Axial Acquisition ("Step & Shoot")

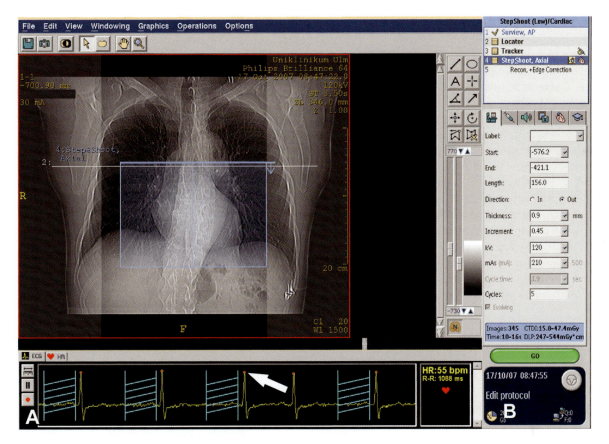

Fig. 8c.7 Limited field of view with "Step & Shoot". The "gray stripes" on both sides of the patient in the scanogram (**Panel A**) reflect the limited field of view (250 mm). To avoid unnecessary radiation exposure an additional lateral scanogram should be obtained only in patients with above-average thoracic diameters. Additionally, prospective ECG triggering with online arrhythmia handling is also shown skipping one RR cycle (*arrow* in **Panel A**). **Panel B** shows the dose indication box, displaying CTDI and DLP values as ranges (e.g., CTDI 15.8–47.4 mGy and DLP 247–544 mGy × cm), where the lowest value represents a case without any arrhythmia, and the highest value a case with severe continuous irregularities. The "Time" field in this box gives the scan time range without irregularities (minimum) and the scan time in the case of continuous irregularities (maximum). The slice increment and thickness are the same as with the helical protocol

scans. These characteristics are reflected in the values that are defined in the dropdown menus for both "Increment," and "Thickness" fields (**Fig. 8c.7**).

8c.2.2 Dose Indication Box

Since the "Step & Shoot" scan time and irradiation profile are not known ahead of time (because of potential online arrhythmia handling), the indication box was changed in comparison to retrospective image acquisition (**Fig. 8c.2**) to reflect this uncertainty (**Fig. 8c.7**).

8c.2.3 Injection Protocol

The injection protocol for "Step & Shoot" acquisition is identical to that used for current helical acquisition. It is important to emphasize the fact that the minimal post-threshold delay is 7 s, since this is the amount of time needed to reach the initial scan position and to build up adequate tube voltage. Another important drawback is that by prospective acquisition, only one cardiac phase can be acquired. The cardiac phase needs to be selected beforehand, and the center of the phase can vary from 40–85% of the RR interval.

8c.3 Reconstruction

Image reconstruction is performed using comparable parameters for retrospectively and prospectively acquired data (**Table 8c.2**), with cardiac standard filters XCA-D during mid-diastole and end-systole of the cardiac cycle (**Fig. 8c.8**). Philips uses an adaptive multisegment reconstruction algorithm integrating 3D voxel-based backward projection of the cone beam. Image reconstruction using the raw data from up to five segments from consecutive cardiac cycles improves the theoretical temporal resolution. A coronary artery will be reconstructed from partial raw data from several consecutive RR intervals. This reconstruction principle is applied separately for each voxel.

Left/right ventricular analysis requires ECG intervals equally spaced by a maximum of 10%. It is advisable to perform an additional reconstruction of the raw data in a lung-adapted window setting using maximum fields of view.

Table 8c.2 Typical reconstruction parameters

	Prospective helical scan	Step & Shoot
Reconstruction filter kernel	Xres Standard (XCA-D)	Xres Standard (XCA-D)
Reconstruction field of view	Approximately 200 mm	Approximately 200 mm
Matrix	512 × 512	512 × 512
Slice thickness	0.9 mm	0.9 mm
Reconstruction increment	0.45 mm	0.45 mm
Reconstructed ECG intervals[a]	Normally 40 and 75%, for functional analysis 0–90% equally spaced by 10%	Normally 75% (40–85%)

[a] Percentages indicate the center of the image reconstruction interval

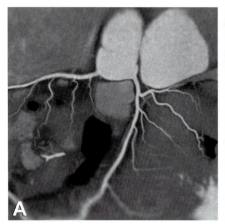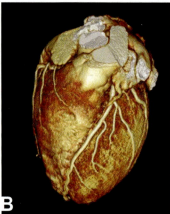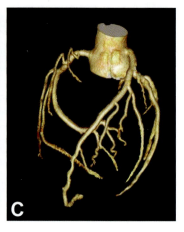

Fig. 8c.8 Reconstructions from a "Step & Shoot" examination: two-dimensional map (**Panel A**), volume-rendering of the heart (**Panel B**), and the extracted coronary tree (**Panel C**) reconstructed at 75% of the R-R cycle using an XCA-D filter

General Electric Light Speed VCT

L. Lehmkuhl

8d.1	Electrode Placement and ECG	93
8d.1.1	Electrode Placement	93
8d.1.2	ECG Monitor	93
8d.2	Scan Preparation	93
8d.2.1	Breathing Instructions	93
8d.2.2	Scout Scans	94
8d.3	Scan Modes, Bolus Timing, and Image Acquisition	95
8d.3.1	CT Coronary Angiography Scan Modes	95
8d.3.2	Bolus Timing	95
8d.3.3	Image Acquisition	97
8d.4	Image Reconstruction	100

Abstract

This chapter describes how CT coronary angiography is performed on General Electric scanners.

8d.1 Electrode Placement and ECG

8d.1.1 Electrode Placement

It is recommended that the electrodes not be placed over muscle, scar tissue, or hair; the proper placement is medially over the clavicle to avoid the muscle tissue when the arms are raised over the head. It is very important to ensure good skin contact. Details of patient preparation for CT coronary angiography on all scanner types are presented in Chaps. 6 and 7.

Figure 8d.1 shows proper lead placement using the IVY ECG monitor: First raise the patient's arms above the head, and then position the leads as shown. Place the two upper leads directly on the patient's clavicle. This placement provides the best signal for the IVY monitor. To avoid incompatibilities, do not use patient monitoring electrodes that may be available from other departments in your facility. The electrodes recommended by General Electric (GE) are Dyna/Trace 1500 by Conmed.

8d.1.2 ECG Monitor

Turn on the ECG machine and make sure that there are good connections to the gantry and leads. A good connection is confirmed if "CONNECTED" appears in the upper right display area of the monitor. Otherwise, check to make sure that the cable connecting the ECG machine to the backside of the gantry is plugged in properly and that the same cable is connected to the ECG machine. In case of low signal, check the electrode placement and choose an alternative position if needed (**Fig. 8d.1**). If there is "noise" within the ECG wave, it is recommended that you do not scan until this condition is corrected.

8d.2 Scan Preparation

8d.2.1 Breathing Instructions

Prior to the scan, have the patient practice the automatic breathing instructions. Scanning is sufficiently rapid that it is not necessary for the patient to hyperventilate. The scanning time should be no longer than 5–8 s on average. Let the patient take one breath in, blow it out, then take a breath in and hold it, while you watch the ECG monitor and take note of the patient's heart rate during breath-holding. A patient who has any difficulty holding his or her breath may be put on 2–4 l min^{-1} of oxygen via a nasal cannula. Oxygen administration may also help to lower the heart rate.

When recording the breathing instructions for cardiac CT that are programmed in the scanner, make sure to give

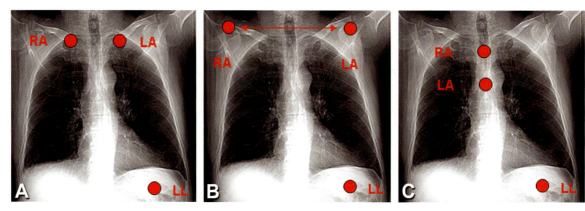

Fig. 8d.1 ECG electrode placement. **Panel A** shows a scanogram depicting the recommended ECG lead placement for best signal clarity. If the signal is low or the QRS peak is not noticeably stronger than the other ECG wave segments, using one of the two alternate positions (**Panels B** and **C**) may improve the ECG signal and its detection

the breathing instructions slowly. The breathing instructions should be no shorter than 10 s. When recording the instructions, and after you say, "take a breath in and hold it," be sure to wait for 3–5 s (of silence) prior to clicking on the "stop recording" button. This delay will give the patient enough time to hold his or her breath before the actual start of the scan and for the heart rate to stabilize; otherwise the patient may still be breathing in during the first several slices, which could lead to motion artifacts on the images.

8d.2.2 Scout Scans

The following steps, summarized in **List 8d.1**, should be performed to choose the correct scan protocol and to acquire the scout scans.

If the heart rate is not displayed on the screen and you have a "red" gating box, the scanner is not reading the patient's waveform. To correct this problem, try the following: (1) click on the red "Gating" box and turn off the gating, then turn it back on; (2) check all connections between the gantry and the ECG machine; and (3) check once again for proper placement of the leads on the patient.

List 8d.1. Choice of protocol and scout acquisition

1. Landmark the patient at the sternal notch
2. Select "new patient" and enter patient data
3. Select the anatomical area (chest)
4. Select the snapshot (cardiac) protocol from the main menu
5. On the scout screen, check to make sure you are in "Active Gating" mode and that the gating is fine, then take the scout views
6. Use the cardiac breathing protocol for the scout scans and all subsequent scans (**Fig. 8d.2**)
7. Monitor the patient's heart rate during the breath-hold[a]
8. When the two scout scans are completed, select "next series" to display the next step of the protocol

[a] The body's natural physiologic response during breath-hold is to reduce the heart rate by approximately 5 beats per min. Knowing what the patient's heart rate does during the breath-hold will help you determine what scanning mode to use during the cardiac scan (**Fig. 8d.3**).

8d.3 • Scan Modes, Bolus Timing, and Image Acquisition

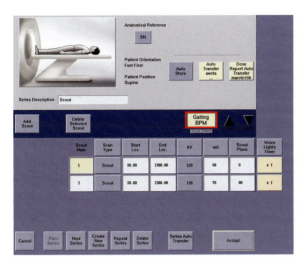

Fig. 8d.2 Planning the scout (scanogram) acquisition. Make sure that "Active Gating" (see *red frame*) has been selected when taking the two scout views (AP and lateral). The cardiac breathing protocol should be used for the scout scans and all subsequent scans

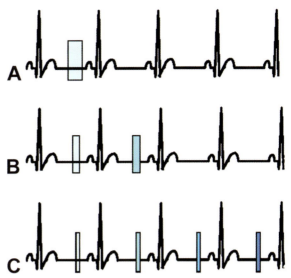

Fig. 8d.3 Alternative retrospective cardiac reconstruction methods. **Panel A** shows the "SnapShot Segment Mode" (halfscan): heart rate, 30–74 beats per min; 1 sector; reconstruction window, 175 ms; a retrospectively gated reconstruction using data from 2/3 of a gantry rotation to create an image from one cardiac cycle. **Panel B** shows the "SnapShot Burst Mode" (multisegment): heart rate, 75–113 beats per min; 2 sectors; reconstruction window, ~87 ms; a retrospectively gated reconstruction using data from up to two cardiac cycles within the same cardiac phase to create an image at a given table/anatomic location. **Panel C** shows the "SnapShot Burst Plus Mode" (multisegment): heart rate, >113 beats per min; 2, 3, or 4 sectors; reconstruction window, 44 ms; stable heart rates; a retrospectively gated reconstruction using data from up to 4 cardiac cycles within the same cardiac phase to create an image at a given table/anatomic location

8d.3 Scan Modes, Bolus Timing, and Image Acquisition

8d.3.1 CT Coronary Angiography Scan Modes

There are three different modes for retrospectively gated reconstruction that can be used for image acquisition, depending on the patient's heart rate. These modes are described in **Fig. 8d.3**. Alternatively, in patients with low and stable heart rates, prospectively ECG-gated (i.e., triggered) axial acquisitions (nonhelical) can also be performed; this approach has the advantage of reducing the radiation exposure.

8d.3.2 Bolus Timing

To calculate the exact arrival time of the contrast medium in the coronary arteries, the test bolus protocol described in **Table 8d.1** is recommended. View the scout and place an axial monitoring scan 1 cm below the carina. If a non-contrast localizer series was previously done (e.g., for calcium scoring), you may also scroll through these images and determine the location for the axial monitoring scan by manually typing the location into the View/Edit screen.

If you have a dual-head injector, it is recommended that you follow the contrast test bolus with a 20-ml saline chaser. Scan the patient with the cardiac breathing protocol and note the heart rate during the scan.

Once all of the test bolus images are reconstructed, highlight the view port in which they are loaded, select the measurement icon on the "Exam Rx Desktop," then select "MIROI" (Multi-Image Region of Interest). Select the elliptic ROI from the pop-up box on the screen, and place the ROI in the ascending aorta and size it to fit completely within the aorta. Then click OK on the pop-up box and calculate the bolus arrival time as described in **Fig. 8d.4**. Click on "Next series" to display the gated cardiac helical acquisition protocol. Enter in the prep delay, based on the test bolus. Alternatively, a bolus tracking technique can be selected by clicking on "Smart Prep." For bolus tracking, a threshold of 120–150 HU is recommended for initiation of the subsequent helical scan (**Fig. 8d.5**).

Table 8d.1 Parameters of the test bolus scan

Parameter	Value
Rotation time	0.5 s
Interval	0
Thickness	5 mm
Prep delay	5 s
Interscan delay	1.5 s
SFOV	Large
DFOV	25 cm
kV	120
mA	40
No. of scans	14
Contrast agent amount	15 ml
Injection rate	5 ml s^{-1}, or the same injection rate as for the cardiac angiogram

DFOV display field of view. This term describes the central part of the scan field of view, which is chosen for image reconstruction. *SFOV* scan field of view. This term describes the maximum diameter of the acquired scan area that can be used for image reconstruction

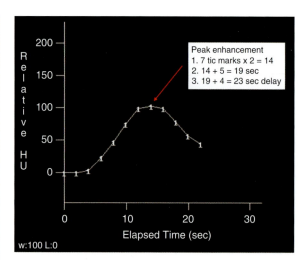

Fig. 8d.4 Time-to-peak curve derived from the test bolus acquisition. On the graph image, count each tic mark on the line graph to the peak of the curve, multiply the number of tic marks by 2, and then add 5 s. Remember that image no. 1 is at 5 s and the tic marks are 2 s apart. This time represents the time it takes for the contrast agent once injected to reach the root of the aorta, where the coronary arteries arise (time-to-peak enhancement). Once you have the time-to-peak enhancement, add an additional 4 s (to allow for filling of the distal coronary vessels); this number is now the pre-scan delay or prep group delay for the cardiac CT exam. In brief, prep delay is calculated as follows: (number of tic marks × 2) + 5 s + 4 s; alternatively, it can be expressed as: peak + 9 s. This bolus time is a key parameter to use for the gated cardiac acquisition.

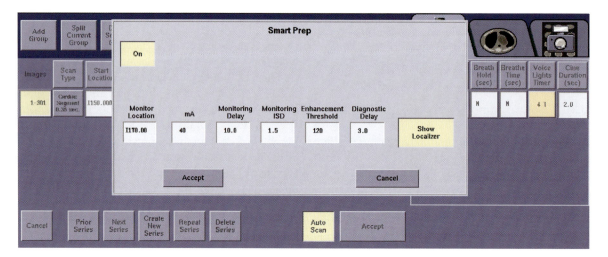

Fig. 8d.5 Choosing the parameters for bolus tracking ("Smart Prep"). An enhancement threshold of 120–150 HU is recommended

8d.3.3 Image Acquisition

Prescribe the location of the scan on the scout using graphic Rx, or type in the start and end locations using explicit Rx, on the basis of the noncontrast localizer images. Use the scan parameters described in **Table 8d.2**. Choose detector coverage, helical thickness, and rotation time as shown in **Fig. 8d.6**.

Just prior to scanning the patient, it is very important to check the ECG trace on the scanner console to make sure that you are properly gating and that the scanner is triggering on the appropriate segment of the ECG wave. You should see a "RED" line on the R peak of the QRS complex on the patient's ECG wave. If you do not see the "RED" line on the R peak but rather somewhere else, make the appropriate adjustments to the electrode placement or monitor settings to ensure proper gating on the R peak. The "white" area represents the reconstruction window of 75% in the RR interval used for the reconstruction of the first set of images. The ECG trace on the console refreshes every 2 s.

Table 8d.2 Image acquisition parameters

Scan Parameter	Value	Comment
Scan type	Cardiac helical	
Rotation time	0.35 s	
Start location	–	Based on the scout scans
End location	–	Based on the scout scans
Coverage	Entire heart	
Slice thickness	0.625 mm	See **Fig. 8d.6**
Slice interval	0.625 mm	No overlap (overlap results in more artifacts)
SFOV	Cardiac large	See **Table 8d.3**
DFOV	25 cm	Adjustable as desired to contain coronaries
mA	See **Table 8d.4** and **Fig. 8d.7** for recommended values (adjust these as appropriate for your clinical needs)	ECG modulation can lead to a dose decrease of up to 50% in low stable heart rates; see **Fig. 8d.8** for further instructions
kVp	120	
Pitch	–	The pitch is automatically set by the software, based on the patient's heart rate
Reconstruction type	Standard	
Cardiac noise reduction filters	C1, C2, or C3	These filters allow dose reductions of up to 30% on top f the ECG modulation dose reduction while preserving image quality

DFOV display field of view; *SFOV* scan field of view

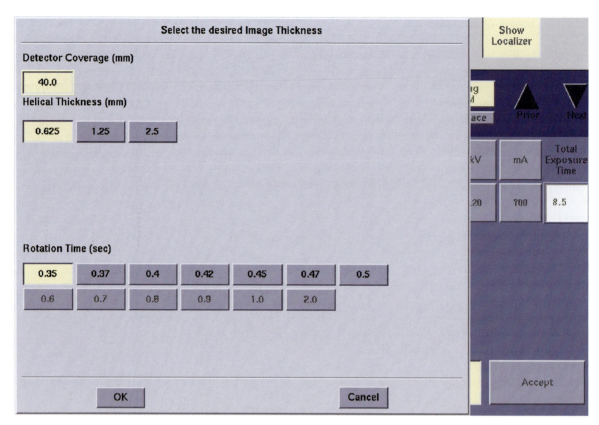

Fig. 8d.6 For cardiac scanning, choose the detector coverage, helical thickness, and rotation time as shown in this screenshot

Table 8d.3 Different cardiac scan fields of view

SFOV	Bowtie filter	DFOV (cm)[a]
Cardiac small	Small	9.6–32
Cardiac medium	Medium	9.6–36
Cardiac large	Large	9.6–50

DFOV display field of view; *SFOV* scan field of view
[a] The standard DFOV for cardiac CT using GE scanners is 25 cm

Table 8d.4 Recommended mA values for ECG modulation

Body weight	Minimum mA value	Maximum mA value
<60 kg (<132 lb)	100	450
60–80 kg (132–176 lb)	250	550
>80 kg (>176 lb)	400	750

If no modulation is desired, the scan should be acquired with the maximum mA value

8d.3 • Scan Modes, Bolus Timing, and Image Acquisition

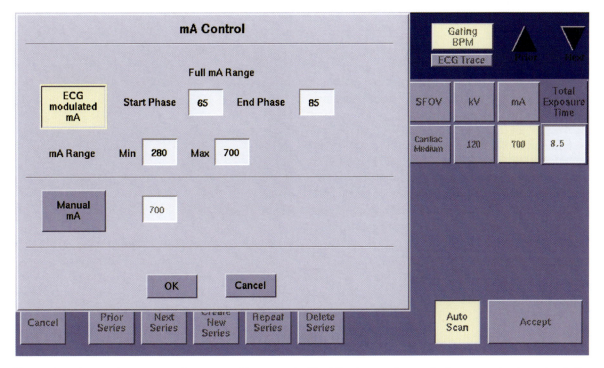

Fig. 8d.7 Adjusting the mA setting for coronary CT angiography. The full mA range phase and mA range can be chosen by clicking on the "mA" button. ECG modulation can be switched off by clicking on the "Manual mA" button. "Min" and "Max" define the mA range of the modulation, whereas "Start phase" and "End phase" describe the part of the RR interval to which the maximum mA is applied. Recommended mA values are listed in **Table 8d.4**

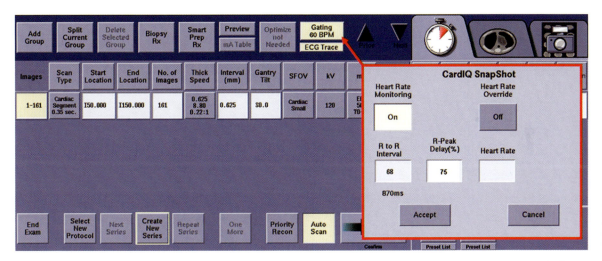

Fig. 8d.8 Before starting the scan, make sure that the reconstruction phase is centered at 75%. The "Heart Rate Override" button allows you to use a lower pitch than suggested by the software

8d.4 Image Reconstruction

Once the scan is completed, select "retro recon." Select the phase button and process the images from 70–80% of the RR interval with an incremental step of 10% in the mode in which the images were acquired. These images (displayed as complete series) will be used if the heart is not frozen at 75% of the RR interval from the initial scan. The images can also be processed from any other point within the RR interval (**Fig. 8d.9**) to make it possible to see images from systole to diastole. If the RCA is not frozen in the 70–80% phase range, it is best to reconstruct the phases centered at 40–55% (end-systole)

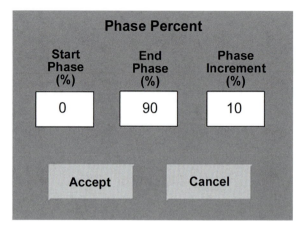

Fig. 8d.9 Reconstruction at different phases

Reading and Reporting

L.J.M. Kroft and M. Dewey

9.1	Reading	101
9.1.1	Selecting Cardiac Phases	101
9.1.2	Systematic Approach	103
9.1.3	Source Images	105
9.1.4	Curved Multiplanar Reformations	107
9.1.5	Maximum-Intensity Projections	114
9.1.6	Volume Rendering and Angiographic Emulation	115
9.1.7	Typical Artifacts	116
9.1.8	Cardiac Function	120
9.2	Reporting	124
9.2.1	Structured Reporting	124
9.2.2	Medical History, Symptoms, and Questions to Be Answered	124
9.2.3	Technical Approach and Image Quality	124
9.2.4	Description of Findings	127
9.2.5	Overall Impression and Recommendations	127
	Recommended Reading	128

Abstract

In this chapter, we describe how to read and report coronary CT angiography studies.

9.1 Reading

9.1.1 Selecting Cardiac Phases

Before starting to read a coronary CT angiography study, it is necessary to select one or more of the reconstructed phases (i.e., "image reconstruction interval") within the cardiac cycle. It is important to select the phase(s) with the sharpest coronary artery depiction to maximize the number of coronary segments rendered without motion artifacts. There are various alternatives for choosing the phases with the best coronary artery image quality, and the optimal method may vary with the scanner used. Since reconstructions with the center of the phase at 80, 70, and 40% of the RR interval are sufficient for image analysis, in most patients, one can automatically reconstruct these phases as predefined intervals and start the analysis by reading these three phases. A second approach is to manually select the best phase by visual inspection of different reconstructions covering the cardiac cycle, but this is a relatively time-consuming method. A third approach that has recently become available is motion mapping, which automatically identifies the end-systolic and mid-diastolic phases with the least overall motion (**Fig. 9.1**). Various automatic phase selection software tools are currently being validated for use in clinical practice. If the phases reconstructed using any of these methods are not sufficient for making a reliable diagnosis, further reconstructions (e.g., from the 10 reconstructions rendered at 10% intervals throughout the RR interval) may be reviewed (**Fig. 9.2**).

However, even after all the desired phases are reviewed, a coronary artery segment may occasionally still prove to be of nondiagnostic quality, e.g., because of artifacts resulting from very high or irregular heart rates or patient movement.

If a stenosis is seen in any phase, this finding should be confirmed by excluding motion artifacts. This confirmation can be accomplished in two ways: (1) by correlating the results with those for the same coronary segment in another phase, and/or (2) by reviewing the axial images in lung window settings in order to detect potential motion in the image (e.g., at the heart–lung border).

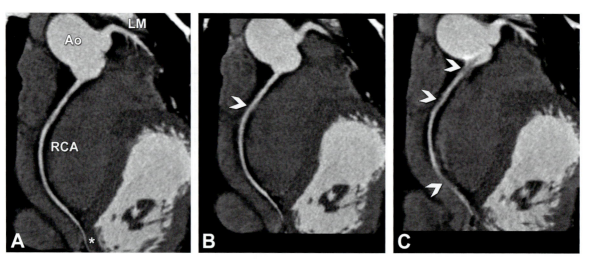

Fig. 9.1 Improved depiction of the right coronary artery (RCA) on curved multiplanar reformations using motion mapping with automatic identification of the phase with least motion during mid-diastole (**Panel A**), when compared with standard reconstructions centered at 70% (**Panel B**) and 80% (**Panel C**) of the cardiac cycle, which show minimal (**Panel B**) and more severe (**Panel C**) motion artifacts (*arrowheads*). Note the excellent visualization of the distal vessel segment with automatic phase selection (*asterisk* in **Panel A**). *Ao* aorta; *LM* left main coronary artery

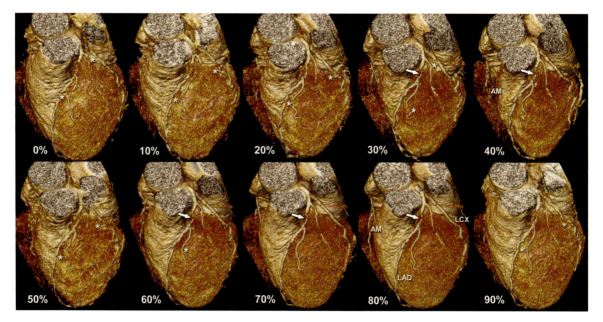

Fig. 9.2 Three-dimensional volume-rendered reconstructions of the coronary arteries (left anterosuperior views) shown for 10 image reconstruction intervals throughout the entire cardiac cycle (centered at 0–90%). There is a significant stenosis (*arrow*) of the proximal left anterior descending coronary artery (LAD), which is best seen at 70 and 80% but also at 40%. In comparison, however, the left circumflex coronary artery (LCX) is best seen at 70 and 80%. There are multiple motion artifacts in the other reconstruction intervals (marked with *asterisks*), rendering these phases nondiagnostic (artifacts were identified using the axial source images). Interestingly, the right coronary artery with its acute marginal (AM) branch is well depicted during mid-diastole (80%) as well as end-systole (40%). In many cases, the right coronary artery is best seen at end-systole (especially at higher heart rates)

9.1.2 Systematic Approach

If no stenoses are seen and image quality is good, it is not necessary to go through all the reconstructed coronary artery phases. The comprehensive assessment of a coronary CT angiography study on a workstation takes time and concentration.

9.1.2 Systematic Approach

The review of a coronary CT angiography data set focuses on the coronary arteries but should also comprise assessment for other cardiac findings and extracardiac findings. As in all radiological examinations, a systematic approach is pivotal to a comprehensive evaluation of all anatomical regions (**List 9.1**). Easy evaluation of the coronary arteries is now possible by reading (semi)automatic curved multiplanar reformations, which are crucial for detecting pathology. However, the findings should always be confirmed on the original slices in axial and/or orthogonal orientations. Reading is improved when curved multiplanar reconstructions and source images can be evaluated simultaneously. Thin-slab (3–5 mm) maximum-intensity projections are usually very helpful in evaluating the continuity of the coronary arteries.

Prestenotic dilatation of the vessel lumen is an interesting indirect indicator of a significant stenosis located distally, and its recognition is critical. Furthermore, aneurysms of the coronary arteries are present in 5% of patients with atherosclerotic coronary artery disease but can also be present in patients without significant stenoses (**Fig. 9.3**).

List 9.1. Systematic approach to reading coronary CT angiography studies[a]

1. Obtain a quick overview of the gross anatomy, e.g., by looking at three-dimensional renderings
2. Assess the individual coronary arteries and major side-branches by using reconstruction tools and viewing original slices, preferably simultaneously[b]
3. Evaluate the cardiac extracoronary structures[c]
4. Evaluate extracardiac organs[d]

---

[a] The approach may vary with the workstation used

[b] Double-oblique orthogonal reconstructions, thin-slab maximum-intensity projections, and curved multiplanar reformation are very helpful displays for evaluating the major coronary arteries and their large side-branches. Any pathology detected on such advanced reconstructions should be confirmed on original axial, coronal, or sagittal slices

[c] This includes the cardiac valves, the myocardium, the atrial, and ventricular cavities (e.g., for presence of intracavitary thrombus), evaluation of (left) ventricular function, the pericardium, and the aortic root

[d] This includes assessment of all organs other than the heart and has to be performed on large fields of view. Evaluate the large vessels (e.g., the aorta for dissection or aneurysm and the pulmonary arteries for presence of emboli), mediastinum, hila, lungs, chest wall and breasts, abdominal organs, and bones

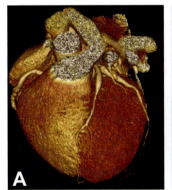 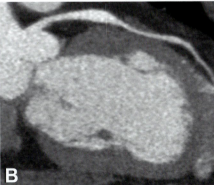 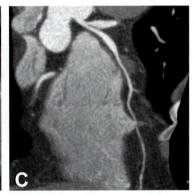

Fig. 9.3 Dilation without significant coronary stenosis. Volume-rendered image (**Panel A**) and multiplanar reconstructions (**Panels B** and **C**) of the left anterior descending coronary artery in a 47-year-old male with atypical chest pain. The patient had no coronary artery stenoses but did have dilating coronary artery disease. Note the dilation in the proximal left descending coronary artery. There is some focal myocardial bridging, and the right and left circumflex coronary arteries were also dilated (not shown)

If images look very poor on every reconstruction despite adequate contrast and compliance of the patient during the examination, one should inspect the recorded ECG tracing for irregularities, such as premature ventricular contraction, extrasystoles, or atrial fibrillation, or search for postprocessing errors by looking at the phases

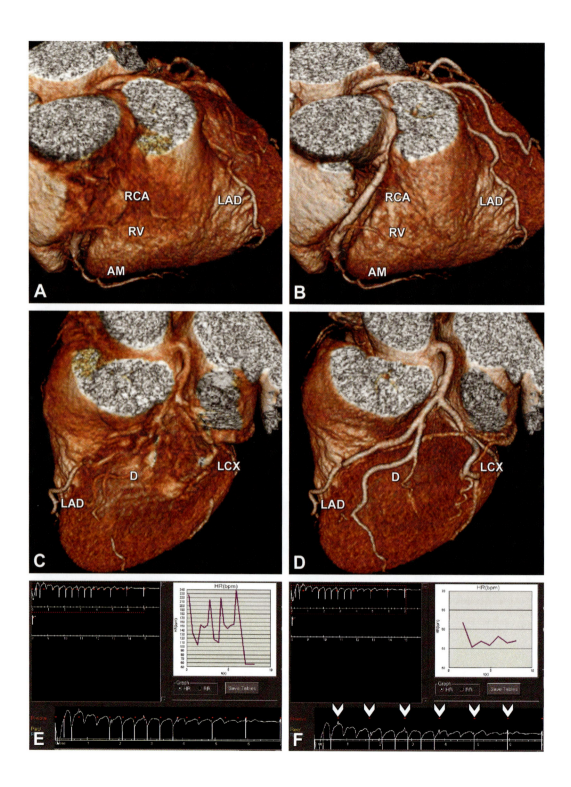

selected for image reconstruction. Using ECG editing, image degradation due to ECG irregularities can often be overcome by deleting or adding R waves for triggering and rereconstructing image data without scanning the patient again (**Fig. 9.4**).

9.1.3 Source Images

Reading coronary CT angiography datasets requires knowledge of coronary and cardiac anatomy (Chap. 3). The axial source images represent the basic reconstructions that contain all information available in the three-dimensional dataset. Conclusions and final diagnoses should always be based on standard slices in the axial and orthogonal planes (which is possible because of isotropic voxel size in CT). Scrolling through the slices back and forth on a workstation is the best way to look at the source images. Additional information can be obtained from thin-slab maximum-intensity projections (see below) and double-oblique positioning of slices along or orthogonal to lesions.

Compared with the source images, all other reconstructions such as curved reformations, maximum-intensity projections, angiographic emulations, and volume rendering (**List 9.2**) tend to reduce the information content and may even obscure relevant information.

> **List 9.2. Reconstructions available for reading coronary CT angiography studies**
>
> 1. Axial, coronal, and sagittal images are the primary source of information
> 2. Curved multiplanar reformations are convenient for identifying stenoses
> 3. Maximum-intensity projections give a good overview of vessels and lesions but may obscure stenoses and overestimate calcified lesions
> 4. Angiographic emulations and three-dimensional renderings may be used for elegant display and presentation of findings

The main advantage of these reconstructions, which can be prepared by the technician, is that they make evaluation of the coronary arteries much easier because large vessel segments are displayed in a single image. This wide view can be beneficial in detecting abnormalities such as short coronary stenoses or wall irregularities (**Fig. 9.5**). Also, reconstructed images can be useful for demonstrating results during multidisciplinary team meetings. Printouts showing the reconstructed coronary arteries can be sent to the referring physicians as summaries of image findings.

Fig. 9.4 Use of ECG editing significantly improves the image quality of reconstructions on the basis of the same raw data (without rescanning the patient). The left side (**Panels A**, **C**, and **E**) shows the results before editing, and the right side (**Panels B** and **D**) the three-dimensional reconstructions obtained after ECG editing. The entire course of the coronary arteries is blurred before ECG editing because of extrasystoles during scanning (**Panel E**, differentiating supraventricular and ventricular extrasystoles was not possible using this data and Holter ECG was recommended). Excluding the arrhythmic peaks and using only the typical R-wave peaks for editing (*arrowheads* in **Panel F**) greatly improves the images of both the right (**Panel B**) and the left (**Panel D**) coronary artery system. The right-hand corner insets in **Panels E** and **F** show the unedited and edited heart rate courses over time that were used for image reconstruction. *AM* acute marginal artery; *D* diagonal branch; *LAD* left anterior descending coronary artery; *LCX* left circumflex coronary artery; *RCA* right coronary artery; *RV* right ventricular branch

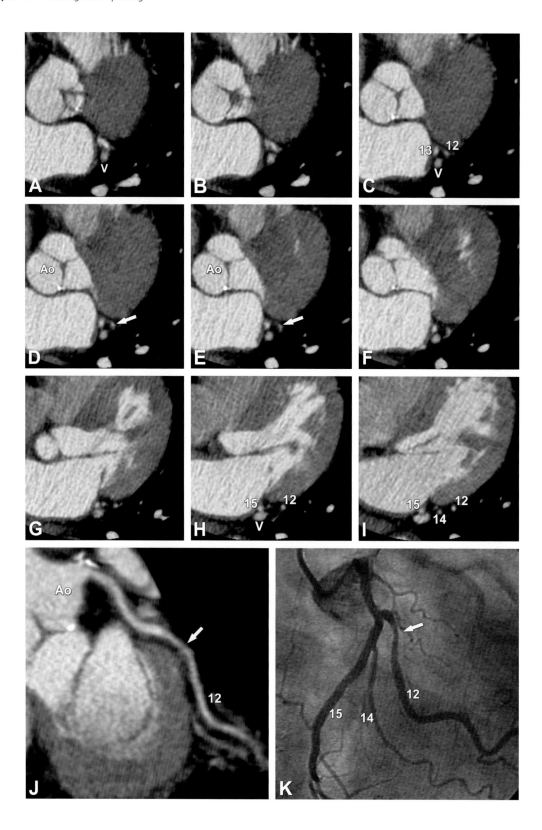

9.1.4 Curved Multiplanar Reformations

Curved multiplanar reformations are generated using a centerline along the coronary vessel path and show large parts of the coronary vessel lumen in a single image (**Figs. 9.5** and **9.6**). Depending on the workstation used, the curved multiplanar reformations may be rotated around their centerlines, thereby rotating the coronary artery lumen around its longitudinal axis and greatly improving the visual estimation of the severity of the stenosis. The curved multiplanar reformations also allow rendering cross-sectional images orthogonal to the vessel course, which further facilitates the quantification of the percent diameter stenosis (based on reference and stenosis diameters, **Fig. 9.7**).

Continuously improving automatic vessel detection and segmentation tools are available for the creation of curved multiplanar reformations. These automatic software tools are currently available on all competitive workstations and allow diagnostic accuracy to be maintained while relevantly reducing analysis time. When using one of the currently available reconstruction tools, however, the user must be aware of two limitations of automatic segmentation that can lead to false-positive or false-negative lesions: First, the automatic vessel probing tools do not always entirely follow the course of the coronary vessels (especially if these are very tortuous). The resulting images may suggest stenoses on the curved multiplanar reformations that are, however, usually readily identified as artifacts (**Fig. 9.8**). The centerline should be checked (e.g., on three-dimensional renderings) when stenoses are suggested (**Fig. 9.8**), and the findings should be confirmed on the original images. The second common limitation of automatic vessel detection is that the most proximal segment of the coronary artery may not be completely probed. Significant proximal stenosis can thus be missed if one looks only at the automatically probed vessel segments. However, this limitation is also easily overcome by manually or automatically adding the vessel portions that have been missed by the automatic tool (**Fig. 9.9**).

In addition to motion artifacts resulting from a rapid or irregular heartbeat, heavily calcified coronary segments pose the greatest challenge because they obscure the coronary artery lumen (**Fig. 9.10**). Heavily calcified segments may not be evaluable, although severe calcifications do not per se exclude evaluation. In this situation, visualization of coronary stenoses can be improved by using specific window-level settings (**Fig. 9.11**).

Fig. 9.5 Short coronary artery stenosis of the first obtuse marginal artery (segment 12) that might be missed on axial images (**Panels A–I**), which show the stenosis on only two consecutive slices (*arrow* in **Panels D** and **E**). In contrast, this 75% diameter stenosis (as measured on quantitative coronary angiography) is easily detected on a curved multiplanar reformation (*arrow* on **Panel J**), demonstrating the advantage of such reconstructions along the vessel course. There is good agreement of the CT finding with conventional coronary angiography (**Panel K**). *V* cardiac vein

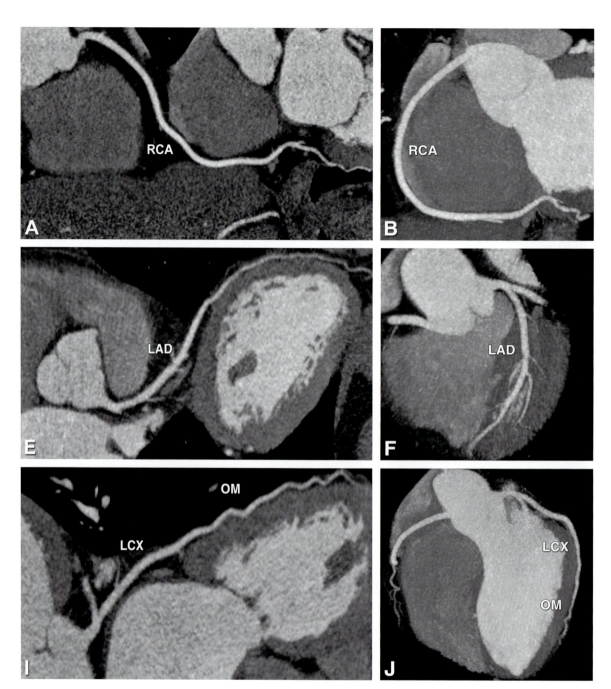

Fig. 9.6 Normal coronary arteries as seen on curved multiplanar reformations (*first column*), maximum-intensity projections (*second column*), and three-dimensional volume-rendered reconstructions (*third column*) of multislice CT using 64 simultaneous detector rows. There is good correlation with conventional coronary angiography (*last column*). The results are shown separately for the right coronary artery (RCA, **Panels A–D**), left anterior descending coronary artery (LAD, **Panels E–H**), and left circumflex coronary artery (LCX, **Panels I–L**). Curved multiplanar reformations allow estimation of the percent diameter stenosis from two perpendicular directions along the long axis or from orthogonal cross-sections and also the detection of coronary artery plaques, with evaluation of their composition. Maximum-intensity projections give a nice overview of the entire vessel but may obscure stenoses because of their projectional nature. Three-dimensional reconstructions provide an overview of long segments of the coronary arteries but should not be used for reading cases. Please note that there is right coronary artery dominance in this patient, with the right coronary giving off the posterior descending artery (PDA), as well as a large right posterolateral artery (RPL, inferior view of the heart in the inset in **Panel C**). *OM* obtuse marginal artery

9.1 • Reading

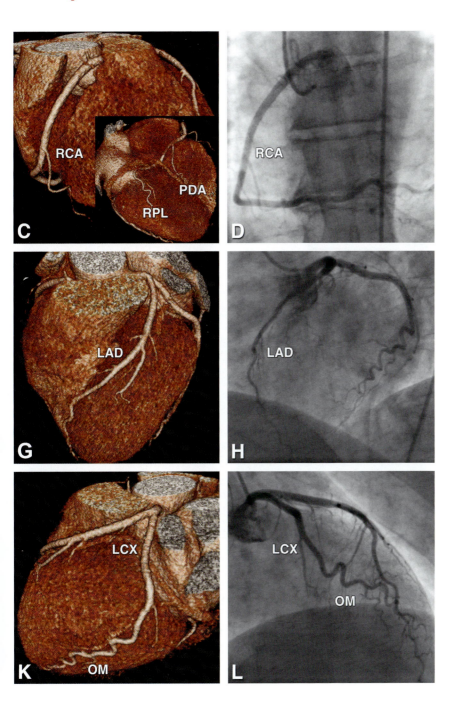

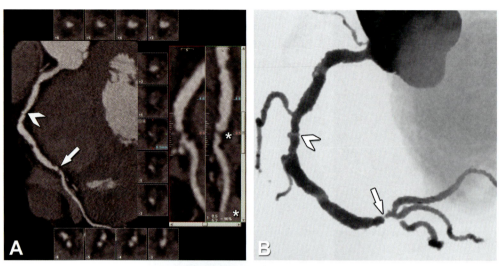
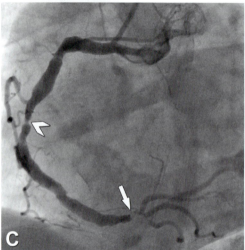

Fig. 9.7 Measurement of percent diameter stenosis using curved multiplanar reformations and orthogonal cross-sections. Right coronary artery with a high-grade stenosis at the crux cordis (*arrow* and *asterisk* in the perpendicular longitudinal views in **Panel A**). The reference vessel diameter is measured proximal and distal to the lesion, and the stenosis diameter is measured within the lesion on orthogonal cross-sections (*squared insets* in **Panel A**). From these measurements (automatic or by caliper) the percent diameter stenosis (in this case 90%) is calculated (*asterisk* in **Panel A**). There is good correlation with angiographic emulation of CT (**Panel B**) and conventional coronary angiography (**Panel C**) regarding this high-grade coronary artery stenosis. A second stenosis is present in segment 2 of the right coronary artery, which was calculated to be a 75% diameter stenosis on quantitative analysis (*arrowhead* in **Panels A–C**)

9.1 · Reading

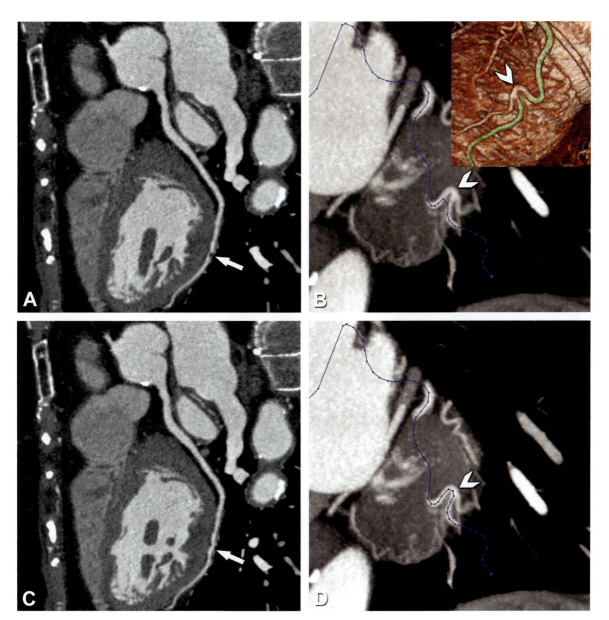

Fig. 9.8 Coronary artery pseudostenosis on a curved multiplanar reformation, caused by an automatic detection tool error. Pseudostenosis on the curved multiplanar reformation along the left circumflex coronary artery (*arrow* in **Panel A**) is caused by a short-track route of the automatic probing tool. This error in vessel tracking (*arrowhead*) is easily recognized on a maximum-intensity projection (*blue centerline* in **Panel B**) and in the *green centerline* on a three-dimensional reconstruction (inset in **Panel B**). After manual correction of the centerline (*arrowhead* in **Panel D**) the curved multiplanar reformation shows the actual course of the left circumflex coronary artery, which is unremarkable and continuous (**Panel C**)

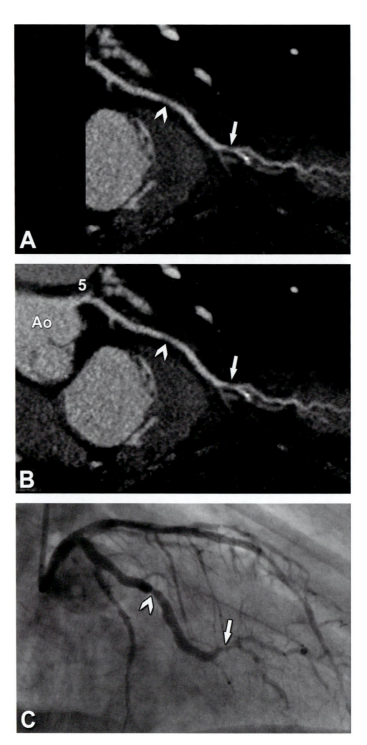

Fig. 9.9 The proximal vessel segment is sometimes missed by the automatic probing tool. Using such a curved reformation (**Panel A**), proximal stenoses cannot be excluded and, as illustrated here, manual extension of the centerline to the aorta (Ao) is necessary to visualize the entire vessel (**Panel B**) including segment 5 (left main coronary artery). There is a nonsignificant (*arrowhead*, 40%) and a significant stenosis in the first obtuse marginal branch (*arrow*, 70%), with good correlation with conventional coronary angiography (**Panel C**)

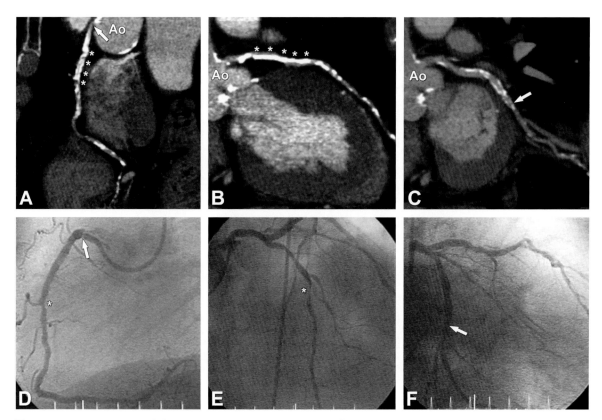

Fig. 9.10 Severe coronary calcifications can hamper the interpretation of CT coronary angiography. In this 82-year-old male patient, there are severely calcified plaques (*asterisks*) along the major course of the right coronary artery (**Panel A**) and left anterior descending coronary artery (**Panel B**). The resulting blooming artifacts obscure the coronary artery lumen, rendering the affected coronary artery segments nondiagnostic. These calcifications were found to cause only short significant stenoses (*asterisk*) in conventional coronary angiography (**Panel D–E**). There are additional less-pronounced calcifications in the left circumflex coronary artery (*arrow* in **Panel C**), but these likewise preclude a definitive diagnosis regarding the presence of significant coronary artery stenosis. Conventional coronary angiography shows moderate stenosis of the left circumflex coronary artery (**Panel F**). Using stent kernels for severely calcified lesions might help to reduce the artifacts, although this approach results in higher noise levels that may also hamper evaluation. Specific window-level settings might be an option for analysis of both calcified and noncalcified plaques (**Fig. 9.11**). Note that there is also a short ostial stenosis of the right coronary artery (*arrow* in **Panels A** and **D**). *Ao* aorta

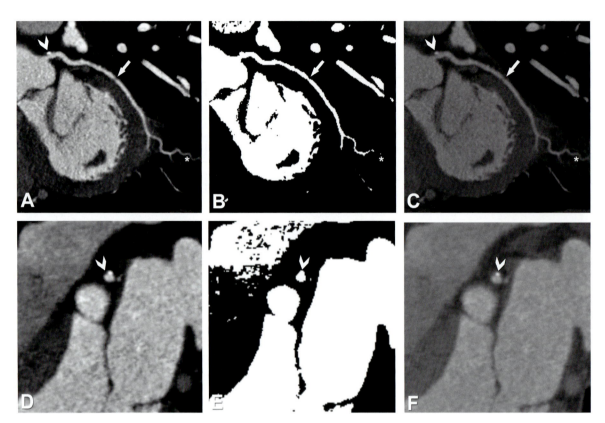

Fig. 9.11 Specific window-level settings may be used for different coronary artery plaques. The *upper row* presents curved multiplanar reformations along the left circumflex coronary artery, and the *lower row* presents cross-sections orthogonal to the left main coronary artery (as indicated by the direction of the *arrowhead* in **Panel A**). Noncalcified coronary plaques and outer vessel boundaries are best visualized using a window representing 155% of the mean density within the coronary lumen and a level representing 65% of the mean density within the lumen as described by Leber et al. (**Panels A** and **D**; this is very commonly equal to 600–700/250–300 HU settings). The noncalcified plaque in the left main coronary artery is nicely seen on the cross-section in **Panel D** (*arrowhead*), and distal vessel segments are depicted on the curved multiplanar reformation using these settings (*asterisk* in **Panel A**). Optimal measurement of the coronary lumen, however, is obtained by keeping the level constant at 65% of the mean lumen density while reducing the window width to 1 (**Panels B** and **E**). Using these settings yields the most accurate measurement of the diameter stenosis in comparison to intravascular ultrasound (in this case 55% diameter reduction) as recently shown by Leber et al. The drawbacks of these settings include the fact that distal vessel segments are not seen as well (*asterisk* in **Panel B**), and calcified plaques are no longer discernible from the lumen (*arrowhead* in **Panel E**). Using more bone-window-like settings (e.g., 1,300/300 HU here), as shown in the last column, reduces the artifacts caused by calcifications and results in less overestimation of calcified coronary plaques than when standard settings are used (*arrowhead* in **Panels C** and **F**)

9.1.5 Maximum-Intensity Projections

Maximum-intensity projections can be varied in projection thickness and give a nice overview of vessel continuity and course in a single image (**Fig. 9.6**). In particular, thin-slab maximum-intensity projections (3–5 mm) are very useful for quickly depicting coronary artery disease. By scrolling through a dataset of thin-slab maximum-intensity projections (e.g., of axial source images), side branches are easily visualized and more side-branches can be recognized than on three-dimensional reconstructions. However, low-grade stenoses may be overlooked. The main drawback of reading maximum-intensity projections is that heavily calcified stenoses present with exaggerated blooming artifacts (**Fig. 9.12**).

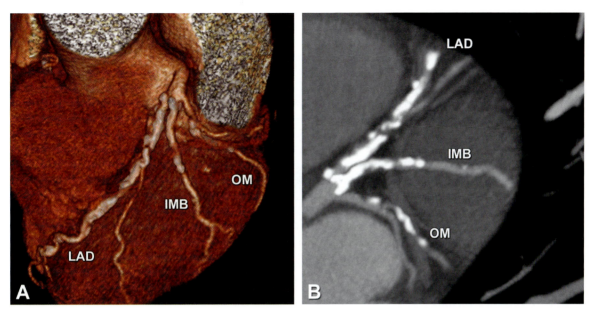

Fig. 9.12 Three-dimensional reconstructions (**Panel A**) and maximum-intensity projections (**Panel B**) do not allow the assessment of severely calcified coronary artery plaques, as shown here in the left anterior descending (LAD), intermediate branch (IMB), and obtuse marginal branch (OM). Because of the projectional nature of maximum-intensity projections, calcified plaques can even be overemphasized (i.e., blooming; **Panel B**). Such blooming artifacts are less pronounced on curved multiplanar reformations and standard two-dimensional images with bone-window-type settings (**Fig. 9.11**). In this patient, conventional coronary angiography revealed significant stenoses in all three vessels

9.1.6 Volume Rendering and Angiographic Emulation

Volume-rendered and angiographic three-dimensional reconstructions are elegant methods for the display and presentation of findings (**Figs. 9.2, 9.4, 9.6, 9.7,** and **9.13**) to referring physicians, patients, and colleagues during interdisciplinary meetings (Chap. 10). Interestingly enough, referring physicians have been reported to prefer angiographic emulations to standard curved

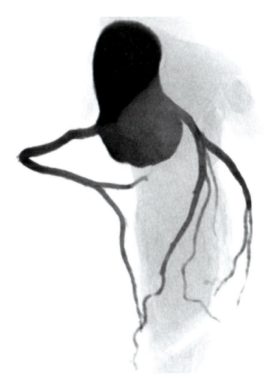

Fig. 9.13 An angiographic emulation of the entire coronary artery tree shows no significant stenoses. The advantage of this type of reconstruction is the striking similarity to conventional angiography, which helps interventionalists rapidly grasp the type and location of coronary lesions before performing invasive procedures. The drawback is that only the lumen and not the underlying plaque is seen on these images (**Fig. 9.7**)

> **List 9.3. The most important artifacts in coronary CT angiography**
>
> 1. Blooming artifacts caused by calcifications
> 2. Motion artifacts causing blurring
> 3. Low-contrast artifacts

multiplanar reformations, while simultaneously identifying the limited visibility and assessability of coronary plaques on these images as a main drawback. Coronary interventionalists may also prefer angiographic emulations of CT data, since they are used to viewing coronary arteries in predefined angiographic projections. Angiographic emulations look much like the interventional angiographic images, and if the desired angled projections are generated, these images may serve as improved anatomic roadmaps for guiding interventions. Making a diagnosis using only three-dimensional reconstructions is not recommended because of the abovementioned limitations.

9.1.7 Typical Artifacts

It is necessary to understand the technical limitations of CT that affect image quality in coronary angiography. The recognition of artifacts that can simulate coronary artery stenoses is particularly critical. The most important artifacts encountered in coronary CT angiography are summarized in **List 9.3**.

Artifacts have major implications for coronary CT angiography. Although spatial and temporal resolution has been greatly improved with the current generation of 64-slice CT scanners when compared with earlier scanners, artifacts are still a major problem. Such artifacts, which generally result from inappropriate motion, can preclude the evaluation of parts of the coronary arteries, as is still the case in 3–12% of coronary artery segments imaged by 64-slice CT scanners. Moreover, artifacts are the main cause of false-positive and false-negative diagnoses regarding the presence of coronary artery stenosis, with misinterpretation being generally attributable to the presence of coronary artery calcifications (**Figs. 9.10** and **9.12**). Other important causes of misinterpretation are motion artifacts and poor contrast-to-noise ratio in obese patients.

Nearly all artifacts in CT are caused by limitations related to spatial resolution, temporal resolution, noise, and the reconstruction algorithms used. Artifacts cause blurring, blooming, streaks, missing data, discontinuities, and poor contrast enhancement.

Spatial resolution is the ability to visualize small structures in the scanned volume and is considered in three dimensions. Important parameters of spatial resolution are voxel size and geometric unsharpness. In the x-y plane, a pixel size of $0.35 \times 0.35\,mm^2$ can be obtained with a reconstructed field of view of 180 mm and a 512^2 pixel matrix. The greatest improvement introduced by the current generation scanners is that volumes with smaller section thickness in the z-axis can be obtained. With 64-slice CT, $64 \times 0.6\,mm$ or $64 \times 0.5\,mm$ collimations are achieved. Geometric unsharpness depends on factors such as focal spot size, detector size, and scanner geometry. Limitations in spatial resolution cause partial volume artifacts as a result of the attenuation coefficient in voxels that are heterogeneous in composition. Resulting artifacts include blooming and blurring, especially in the presence of calcifications (**Figs. 9.10** and **9.12**).

Temporal resolution is the ability to resolve rapidly moving objects and is strongly related to coronary artery size and motion. With the ECG-synchronized scanning techniques and rapid rotation times available today, it is possible to obtain "frozen" images by using half-scan or adaptive multisegment reconstruction at the cardiac phase with the least motion. If the cardiac rest phase is shorter than the scanner's image reconstruction window, motion artifacts occur, but images usually still have adequate diagnostic quality if the artifacts are slight (**Fig. 9.1**). Depending on the heart rate, image quality is generally best in diastole or at late systole (**Fig. 9.2**). Overall, image quality is better in patients with low and stable heart rates. For this reason, beta blocker administration is recommended to lower and stabilize the heart rate. For heart rates <65 beats per min, image quality is usually best at mid-diastole, whereas for heart rates >75 beats per min, the best image quality shifts to systole. At low heart rate, a single time-phase reconstruction is usually enough to visualize all the coronary artery segments with diagnostic quality. At high heart rates, additional reconstructions may be necessary. In conclusion, limitations in temporal resolution cause blurring that may hamper the coronary artery evaluation. The smaller the coronary artery size the greater the effect of motion on the diagnostic image quality.

Respiratory motion can seriously degrade the image quality (**Fig. 9.14**). With scan times of 8–12 s on current 64-slice CT scanners, patients are usually able to hold their breath during scanning.

Image noise is mainly dependent on the number of photons used to make the image. Large chest sizes result in higher image noise, which can be reduced by adjusting the dose settings (kV, mA) to account for the patient's size (Chaps. 7 and 8). Contrast is improved by using

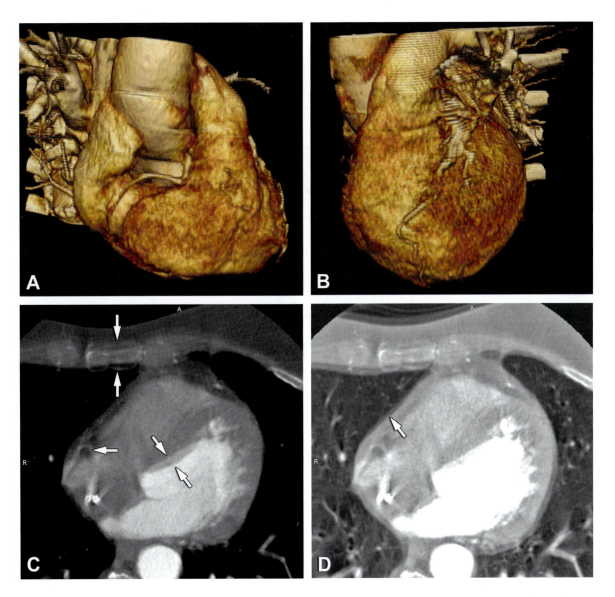

◘ **Fig. 9.14** Severe respiratory motion artifacts. Volume-rendered images (**Panels A** and **B**) and axial source images using soft tissue setting (**Panel C**) and lung window-level setting (**Panel D**) in a 46-year-old female patient who panicked during contrast agent injection and was then unable to hold her breath during scanning. The right coronary artery (**Panel A**) and left coronary artery (**Panel B**) were not evaluable. Note the motion visible in the area of the sternum, right coronary artery, and interventricular septum (*arrows* in **Panel C**). Breathing is also clearly indicated by blurring of the vascular structures and cardiac double contour in the lung setting (*arrow* in **Panel D**). Note that the coronary arteries are not well visualized (**Panels A–C**). The movement of body structures due to breathing resulted in a nondiagnostic scan

iodinated contrast agents. Other influencing factors are the kV setting used and whether patients are adequately instructed on how to hold their breath. (The Valsalva maneuver should be avoided because it impairs contrast agent flow to the heart.) At the workstation, window-level settings can optimize image contrast. Artifacts caused by noise and contrast-to-noise limitations result in poor overall image quality (high noise-level images) and images with low contrast (**Fig. 9.15**).

Reconstruction algorithms also cause artifacts. Spiral acquisition may cause geometric distortion, resulting in dark shadows near the coronary arteries that should

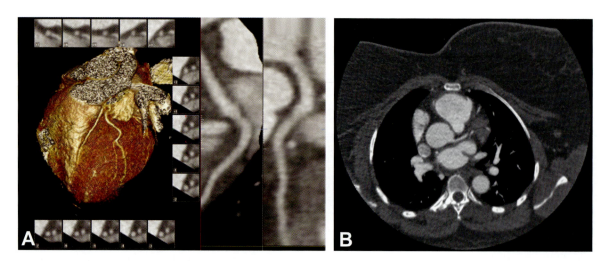

Fig. 9.15 Issues with high noise levels. A volume-rendered image with curved multiplanar reformations (**Panel A**) and axial source images using soft tissue setting (**Panel B**) in a 65-year-old very obese female patient. The image is noisy and of moderate quality despite the use of higher kV and mA settings (135 kV and 350 mA) to increase the radiation dose. Only the proximal parts of the coronary arteries can be evaluated well. Compare the image quality in **Panel A** with that of other figures (e.g., **Fig. 9.6**). Small side-branches are not visible in this overweight patient

not be confused with noncalcified plaques (**Fig. 9.16**). Other artifacts related to limitations in reconstruction algorithms are beam-hardening artifacts (e.g., resulting from high-density contrast agent injection) causing dark bands, as well as metal objects causing complex artifacts, including beam-hardening and partial-volume artifacts (**Fig. 9.17**). Fully automated reconstruction tools used during postprocessing can also result in image artifacts (**Figs. 9.8** and **9.9**). An irregular heart rate during scanning, such as that resulting from premature atrial con-

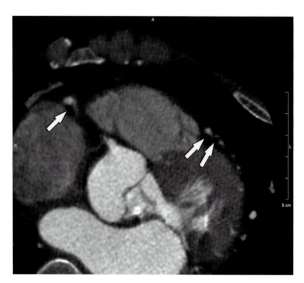

Fig. 9.16 Artifacts resulting from coronary artery motion and geometric distortion appear as *dark spots* adjacent to the right coronary artery and the left anterior descending coronary artery, including its diagonal branches (*arrows*). These artifacts should not be confused with noncalcified coronary artery plaques

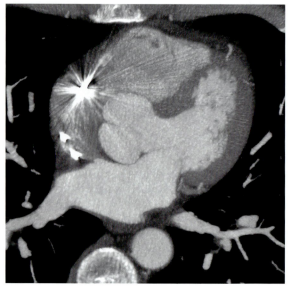

Fig. 9.17 Beam-hardening artifacts in a patient with a pacemaker lead (metal artifact) obscuring the right coronary artery. The patient had no coronary artery stenosis. Note the dilated aortic root with a maximum size of 4.7 cm

9.1 · Reading

traction, can lead to erroneous phase selection during that abnormal heart beat, which may cause blurring or even pseudostenosis (**Fig. 9.18**). We recommend checking the ECG during image interpretation to recognize heart rate irregularities that may cause these types of artifacts, which can be eliminated by manual ECG editing (**Figs. 9.4** and **9.18**). If pathology such as coronary artery stenosis is identified on postprocessed images, the findings should always be confirmed by reviewing the original data set (axial and/or orthogonal source images).

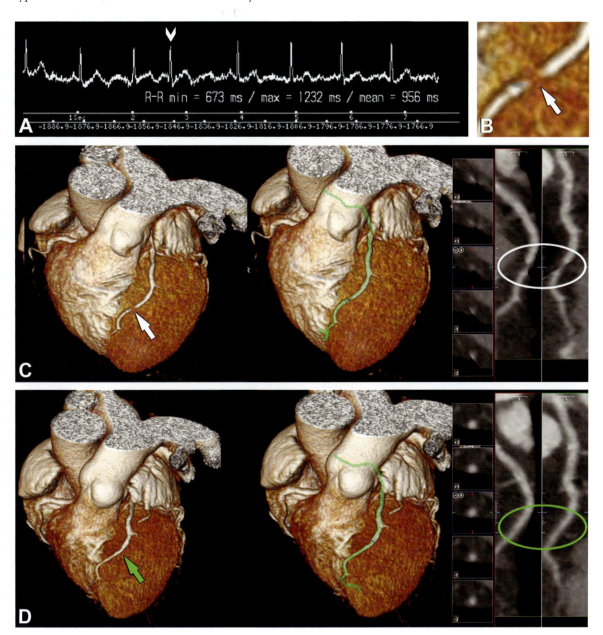

Fig. 9.18 Artifacts caused by irregular heart rate during scanning. CT coronary angiography in a 73-year-old female patient with suspected acute coronary artery syndrome. Premature atrial contraction after the third R-peak (*arrowhead*), followed by a compensatory long pause before the next R-peak (**Panel A**). Automatic reconstruction centered at 75% of the RR interval was performed with suboptimal time points relative to the R-peaks at the location of the short RR interval, giving rise to a coronary artery pseudostenosis (*arrow* in **Panels B** and **C**). Reconstruction at an optimal time point (ECG editing) resulted in normal image quality and elimination of the pseudostenosis (*green arrow* and *circle* in **Panel D**)

9.1.8 Cardiac Function

In addition to the location and severity of coronary artery stenoses and the presence of diabetes mellitus, left ventricular ejection fraction (above vs. below 50%) is of pivotal importance in determining the most suitable therapy for patients (percutaneous coronary intervention vs. coronary artery bypass grafting, **Fig. 9.19**). Also, left ventricular ejection fraction has been shown to be the most important prognostic factor for cardiac events and death that can be derived from diagnostic testing. Cardiac function analysis is routinely performed as part of CT analysis on workstations, using automatic or semiautomatic software tools (**Fig. 9.20** and **9.21**). These software tools make it possible to manually change the contours if the automatically detected contours are not sufficiently accurate. Quantitative analysis of regional cardiac function is

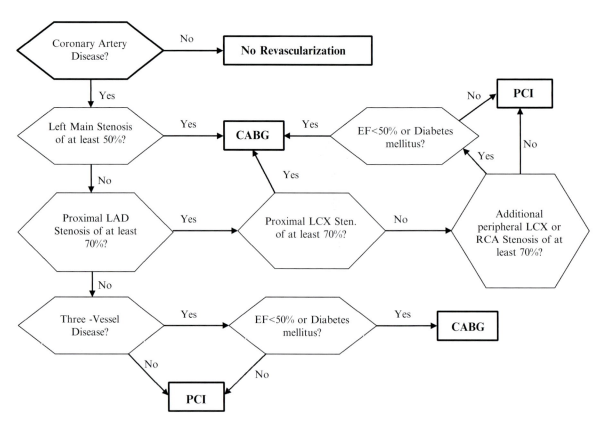

Fig. 9.19 Flowchart for the management of patients with suspected coronary artery disease, according to current guidelines. Interventional treatment is indicated when the percent diameter stenosis is at least 70%, or 50% for the left main coronary artery. Whether coronary artery bypass grafting (CABG) or percutaneous coronary intervention (PCI) should be performed is influenced by the presence of left main disease or left main equivalents as well as global left ventricular cardiac function (ejection fraction, EF) and the presence or absence of diabetes mellitus. This situation highlights the importance of locating coronary stenoses and assessing left ventricular global cardiac function by CT. The guidelines on which this flowchart is based were established by the American College of Cardiology/American Heart Association for conventional coronary angiography: (1) "For the Management of Patients With Chronic Stable Angina" (Gibbons et al. Circulation 2003), (2) "Update for Coronary Artery Bypass Graft Surgery" (Eagle et al. Circulation 2004), and (3) "For Percutaneous Coronary Intervention" (Smith et al. J Am Coll Cardiol 2001). Recommendations I and Level of Evidence A and B were included in creating the flowchart. *LAD* left anterior descending coronary artery; *LCX* left circumflex coronary artery; *RCA* right coronary artery; With permission from H. Hoffmann et al. Acad Radiol 2007

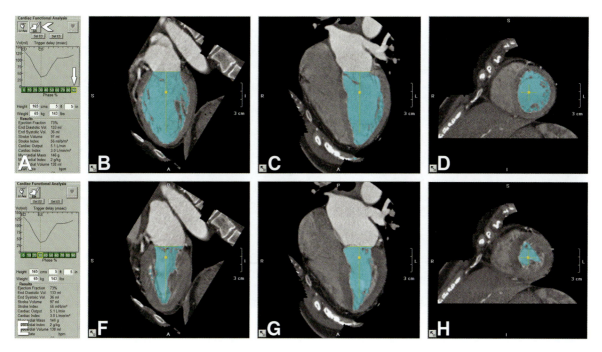

Fig. 9.20 Fully automated cardiac function analysis software (Vitrea, Vital Images). Diastolic frames are shown in the *upper row* (**Panels A–D**) and systolic frames in the *lower row* (**Panels E–H**). This software tool automatically identifies the cardiac axes with the two-chamber (**Panels B and F**) and four-chamber view (**Panels C and G**) as well as the cardiac short axis (**Panels D and H**). The orientation of the left ventricular cardiac axis (marked in *yellow*) and the level at the border of the left atrium and left ventricle can be manually changed. The left ventricular blood pool (excluding the papillary muscles) is also automatically identified and marked in *light blue*. Using the edit function (*arrowhead* in **Panel A**) makes it possible to manually change the automatically defined endo- and epicardial contours in the short-axis views. The end-diastolic time frame is mostly centered around 90% or 0% of the cardiac cycle (**Panel A**, *arrow* at 90%), whereas the end-systolic time frame is mostly at 30 or 40% (**Panel E**). Analysis of 10 image reconstruction intervals serves to calculate a left ventricular volume curve over time (**Panels A** and **E**). Ejection fraction, end-diastolic and end-systolic volumes, stroke volume, and myocardial mass are calculated automatically (**Panels A** and **E**). If the patient's weight and height and the heart rate are given, the software will also calculate stroke index, cardiac index, cardiac output, and myocardial index (**Panels A** and **E**)

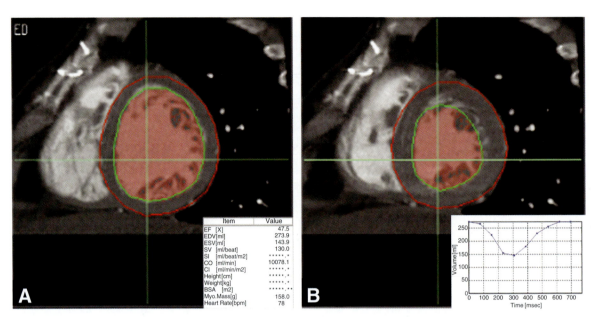

Fig. 9.21 Semiautomatic cardiac function analysis software (Toshiba) with a short-axis slice at end-diastole (**Panel A**) and end-systole (**Panel B**). The *green* and *red contours* in these images represent the automatically generated endo- and epicardial contours, respectively. Note that not all of the area surrounded by the *green line* is assigned to the left ventricular volume, as only pixels with a certain manually adjustable minimum Hounsfield unit density are recognized as part of the blood pool (colored *pink* in the images). In this way, the papillary muscles are excluded from the blood pool. In the inset in **Panel A**, the results of global left ventricular function analysis are displayed; the inset in **Panel B** shows a volume curve, with end-diastole and end-systole represented by the largest and smallest left ventricular volumes, respectively. This semiautomatic analysis tool, although not optimized for this purpose, is also easier to use for right ventricular function assessment than the current fully automated approaches

facilitated by using bull's eye plots, which are available on many workstations (**Fig. 9.22**). Another convenient approach is to evaluate regional cardiac function by looking at cardiac short-axis and long-axis views in cine mode (using 10 reconstructions throughout the cardiac cycle). The cine mode is also useful for the assessment of cardiac valves in different orthogonal or long-axis views (**Figs. 9.23** and **9.24**).

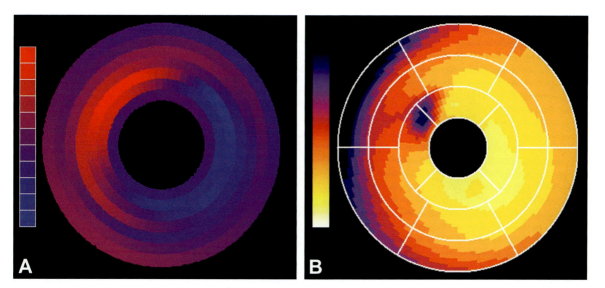

Fig. 9.22 Regional quantitative cardiac function analysis using bull's eye plots of cine magnetic resonance imaging (**Panel A**) and multislice CT (**Panel B**) in a patient with regional hypokinesia in the apical anteroseptal segments (segments 13 and 14, see Chap. 3). This regional wall motion deficit is identified by an analysis of relative wall thickening during systole, and is easily identified by the coloring (*red* in **Panel A** and *dark blue* in **Panel B**), which is different from that of normal segments. In CT (**Panel B**), the borders of the myocardial segments are used as an overlay to facilitate the assignment of findings

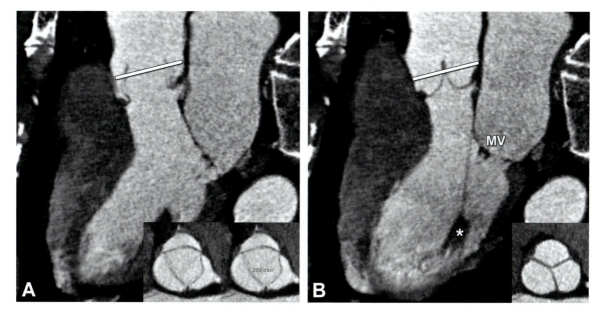

Fig. 9.23 Assessment of the aortic valve using CT in a long-axis three-chamber view during systole (**Panel A**) and diastole (**Panel B**). In this patient, the aortic leaflets are unremarkable; in particular there are no calcifications. During systole, the aortic valve area measures over 3.5 cm^2 (see insets in **Panel A**, which are oriented along the *white line* in **Panel A**). During diastole there is complete closure of the aortic valve leaflets (**Panel B**), and there is no aortic regurgitation area visible (inset in **Panel B**). Note the closed aortic leaflets showing the Mercedes-Benz sign in this inset. *Asterisk* papillary muscles; *MV* mitral valve

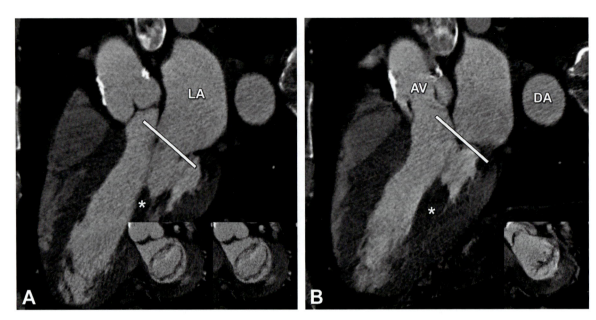

Fig. 9.24 Assessment of the mitral valve in a long-axis three-chamber view during mid-diastole (**Panel A**) and mid-systole (**Panel B**). In this patient, the mitral valve leaflets are unremarkable; in particular there are no calcifications. During mid-diastole, the mitral valve area measures over 6 cm^2 (see insets in **Panel A**, which are oriented along the *white line* in **Panel A**). During systole there is complete closure of the mitral valve (**Panel B**), and there is no mitral regurgitation area visible (inset in **Panel B**). Please note the calcifications of the ascending aorta. *Asterisk* papillary muscles; *AV* aortic valve; *DA* descending aorta; *LA* left atrium

---

List 9.4. Pivotal elements of a coronary CT report[a]

1. Clinical history, symptoms, and question to be answered[b]
2. Technical details of the CT protocol used and image quality
3. Description of findings
4. Overall impression and recommendations for further testing if necessary

[a] The elements are basically the same as for general radiological (CT) reports
[b] To explain why an examination with radiation exposure was necessary

Examples of reports of coronary CT angiography studies are shown in **Figs. 9.25** and **9.26**.

9.2 Reporting

9.2.1 Structured Reporting

Reports of coronary CT angiography studies should be precise and concise. Using a structured reporting technique ensures that no important aspects are overlooked. The important elements of a coronary CT angiography report are summarized in **List 9.4**.

In 2006, the American College of Radiology (ACR) published a practice guideline (Jacobs et al. J Am Coll Radiol 2006) on the conduct and interpretation of cardiac CT studies. This guideline describes how cardiac CT studies should be interpreted and the findings documented. Another, more general ACR practice guideline (Kushner et al. J Am Coll Radiol 2005) describes the steps involved in reporting and communicating diagnostic imaging findings.

9.2.2 Medical History, Symptoms, and Questions to Be Answered

Only the pertinent facts are stated. The question to be answered by the CT investigation should be included (e.g., "coronary artery disease?"). Also relevant are the patient's symptoms (such as angina, dyspnea, fatigue), risk factors for coronary artery disease, history of previous revascularization therapies, and results of prior ischemia testing.

9.2.3 Technical Approach and Image Quality

The report should state the detector collimation, the acquisition method (retrospective [ECG gating] or

9.2 · Reporting

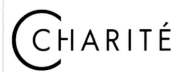 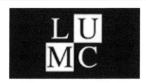

Coronary CT Angiography

History:

- Suspected coronary disease, atypical angina pectoris, equivocal stress ECG

Technique:

Multislice computed tomography with ECG-gated acquisitions through the heart after IV bolus injection of 80 ml of Xenetix 350 in multislice technique (64*0.5 mm slices). Premedication with 1.2 mg sublingual nitroglycerin and an intravenous beta blocker (10 mg Beloc Zok). Retrospective reconstruction using adaptive multisegment reconstruction at 10 time points (0-90%) at 10% intervals throughout the cardiac cycle. 3D and MPR postprocessing at 80% of the cardiac cycle.

Findings:

Very good image quality. Right coronary artery dominance.

LMA: No significant stenoses or plaques.

LAD: No significant stenoses or plaques.

LCX: No significant stenoses or plaques.

RCA: No significant stenoses or plaques.

Left ventricular EF 62.9; EDV, 113.2; ESV, 42.0; SV, 71.2; MM, 131.4 g. No regional akinesia.

Unremarkable appearance of the regions of the lungs visualized.

Overall impression:

Based on this CT of the heart, significant coronary stenosis can be excluded (images and CD attached). Normal left ventricular function.

Fig. 9.25 Example of a report of a coronary CT angiography study in a patient in whom no significant stenoses were found and cardiac function was normal

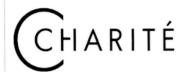 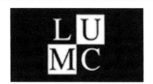

Coronary CT Angiography

History:

- Status post MI 20 years earlier, no angina pectoris, hypertension; obesity; nuclear stress test: anterior ischemia and posterior infarction; exercise ECG: normal; no invasive tests; coronary artery stenosis?

Technique:

Multislice computed tomography with ECG-gated acquisitions through the heart after IV bolus injection of 80 ml of Xenetix 350 in multislice technique (64*0.5 mm slices). Premedication with 1.2 mg sublingual nitroglycerin and an intravenous and oral beta blocker (100 mg Esmolol and 50 mg Atenolol). Retrospective reconstruction using adaptive multisegment reconstruction at 10 time points (0-90%) at 10% intervals throughout the cardiac cycle. 3D and MPR postprocessing at 40 and 70% of the cardiac cycle.

Findings:

Good image quality. Balanced coronary distribution.
LMA: Noncalcified plaque (HU: 15; vol : 32 mm^3). Extends to proximal LAD (segment 6), where it causes significant stenosis.
LAD: Significant stenosis 12 mm in length in segment 6 (60% diameter reduction) due to a noncalcified plaque (HU: 38; vol.: 42 mm^3). Additional noncalcified and nonsignificant (30%) stenosing plaque (HU: 38; vol.: 7 mm^3) in segment 7.
LCX: Noncalcified plaque (HU: 33; vol.: 48 mm^3) in segment 11 without significant stenosis. Segment 13 shows subtotal occlusion (about 95% proximally) due to a noncalcified plaque (HU: 35; vol.: 16 mm^3).
RCA: Reliable evaluation down to the distal portion of segment 2: no significant stenosis. There are two motion artifacts affecting the proximal portion of segment 3, which degrade evaluation of a segment of about 10 mm. No stenoses and plaques further downstream.
Unremarkable appearance of the regions of the lungs visualized.
Left ventricular myocardial function: EF, 35; EDV, 113; ESV, 73; SV, 40; MM, 118 g. Global hypokinesia, posteromedial akinetic areas (segment 10) after history of posterior MI.

Overall impression:

2-vessel coronary artery disease with significant stenoses in segments 6 (LAD) and 13 (LCX) (see attached images). The stenosis in the proximal LAD is very likely responsible for the anterior ischemia found on nuclear imaging. 10 mm long nondiagnostic (unevaluable) portion of segment 3 of the right coronary artery. Reduced left ventricular EF in the presence of marked global hypokinesia and posterior akinesia. Invasive coronary angiography recommended.

prospective [ECG triggering]), the amount and type of contrast agent used, and the doses of nitroglycerin or beta blocker given. One may also add which coronary artery reconstruction phase was used for analysis because doing so will facilitate comparison with future examinations. However, this kind of information may also be stored elsewhere (e.g., in the radiology-information and/or picture archiving and communication system) instead of in the clinical report. It should be stated in the report whether nondiagnostic (not evaluable) coronary artery segments and/or artifacts were present that may have limited the interpretation.

9.2.4 Description of Findings

If one is comparing two studies, this is the best place in a report to mention to which examination the current findings are being compared (e.g., "compared to the prior coronary CT of December 15, 2007"). The coronary artery dominance type (right, left, codominant) should be mentioned. If stenoses or plaques are present, it is critical to provide the location (ostial, near side-branch) and/or segment name or number. Also, the estimated percentage stenosis (**Fig. 9.7**) should be given. As the characteristics of coronary stenoses may determine the success rate of percutaneous coronary interventions, it may be helpful to provide details regarding the length of a stenosis and its eccentricity as well as the presence of calcification or thrombus (**Fig. 9.27**). Further characteristics (e.g., plaque volume, Hounsfield units) may be given as well.

Other cardiac findings such as global and regional cardiac function should be reported if imaging data have been acquired over the entire cardiac cycle. Further cardiac evaluation should include an evaluation of the myocardial tissue, cardiac chambers, and pericardium. Myocardial perfusion defects or other structural myocardial abnormalities, thrombi, and valve-leaflet or annulus calcifications should be described if present. Extracardiac abnormalities in the lungs, bones, chest wall, mediastinum, etc. should be reported. If the portion of the lungs that is visualized is unremarkable, the report should say so. Extracardiac findings are frequently encountered and may explain the patient's chest pain and/or dyspnea, e.g., in the case of incidentally found large diaphragmatic hernia, pulmonary embolism, or emphysema.

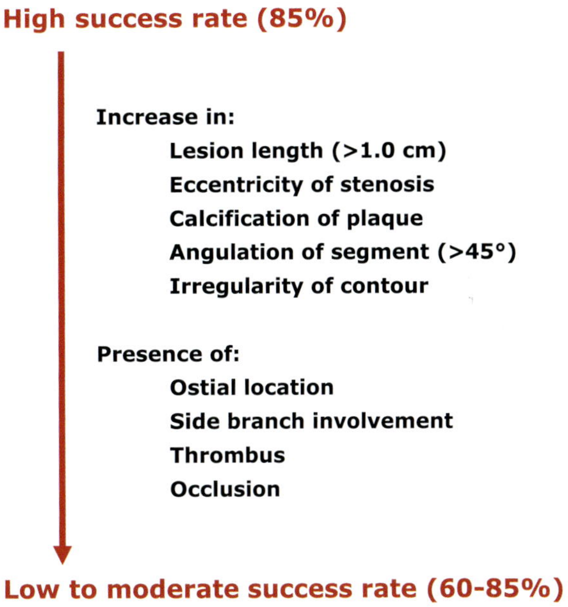

High success rate (85%)

Increase in:
- Lesion length (>1.0 cm)
- Eccentricity of stenosis
- Calcification of plaque
- Angulation of segment (>45°)
- Irregularity of contour

Presence of:
- Ostial location
- Side branch involvement
- Thrombus
- Occlusion

Low to moderate success rate (60-85%)

Fig. 9.27 Influence of different coronary artery stenosis characteristics on the success rate of percutaneous coronary interventions (based on and modified from data provided in Ryan et al. J Am Coll Cardiol 1988 and Smith et al. J Am Coll Cardiol 2001). Success rates may be as low as 60% in patients with very long coronary lesions (>3.0 cm), lesions with severe angulation (>90°), or occlusions existing for more than 3 months. Other important characteristics that can be nicely evaluated with coronary CT are the eccentricity of the stenosis, degree of calcification, and presence of ostial or bifurcation lesions

9.2.5 Overall Impression and Recommendations

The major findings regarding coronary artery stenoses (e.g., "2-vessel coronary artery disease with significant stenoses in. ..."), ventricular function, and relevant cardiac and extracardiac findings should be summarized and the differential diagnoses listed. If the relevance of stenoses appears uncertain, one may recommend which test is indicated next (e.g., nuclear or any other ischemia test to further analyze a borderline stenosis). However, only further investigations that promise to be truly helpful are worth listing here. In case of extracardiac findings, it can be stated whether or not these findings might explain the patient's complaints.

Fig. 9.26 Example of a report of a coronary CT angiography study in a patient in whom significant coronary stenoses were found. Global and regional left ventricular function were also markedly reduced. Plaque volume and density measurement results are given here as an example to illustrate how they can be reported. Note that it is not generally necessary to report coronary plaque findings in such detail

Recommended Reading

1. Bonow RO, Carabello B, de Leon AC, et al. ACC/AHA Guidelines for the Management of Patients With Valvular Heart Disease. Executive Summary. A report of the American College of Cardiology/American Heart Association Task Force on Practice Guidelines (Committee on Management of Patients With Valvular Heart Disease). J Heart Valve Dis 1998; 7:672–707
2. Califf RM, Mark DB, Harrell FE, Jr., et al. Importance of clinical measures of ischemia in the prognosis of patients with documented coronary artery disease. J Am Coll Cardiol 1988; 11:20–6
3. Chin S, Ong T, Chan W, et al. 64 row multi-detector computed tomography coronary image from a centre with early experience: first illustration of learning curve. J Geriatr Cardiol 2006; 3:29–34
4. Coakley FV, Liberman L, Panicek DM. Style guidelines for radiology reporting: a manner of speaking. AJR Am J Roentgenol 2003; 180:327–8
5. de Roos A, Kroft LJ, Bax JJ, Geleijns J. Applications of multislice computed tomography in coronary artery disease. J Magn Reson Imaging 2007; 26:14–22
6. Dewey M, Müller M, Eddicks S, et al. Evaluation of global and regional left ventricular function with 16-slice computed tomography, biplane cineventriculography, and two-dimensional transthoracic echocardiography: comparison with magnetic resonance imaging. J Am Coll Cardiol 2006; 48:2034–44
7. Dewey M, Schnapauff D, Laule M, et al. Multislice CT coronary angiography: evaluation of an automatic vessel detection tool. Fortschr Röntgenstr 2004:478–83
8. Eagle KA, Guyton RA, Davidoff R, et al. ACC/AHA 2004 guideline update for coronary artery bypass graft surgery: a report of the American College of Cardiology/American Heart Association Task Force on Practice Guidelines (Committee to Update the 1999 Guidelines for Coronary Artery Bypass Graft Surgery). Circulation 2004; 110:e340–437
9. Feuchtner GM, Dichtl W, Friedrich GJ, et al. Multislice computed tomography for detection of patients with aortic valve stenosis and quantification of severity. J Am Coll Cardiol 2006; 47:1410–7
10. Feuchtner GM, Dichtl W, Schachner T, et al. Diagnostic performance of MDCT for detecting aortic valve regurgitation. AJR Am J Roentgenol 2006; 186:1676–81
11. Friedman PJ. Radiologic reporting: the hierarchy of terms. AJR Am J Roentgenol 1983; 140:402–3
12. Gibbons RJ, Abrams J, Chatterjee K, et al. ACC/AHA 2002 guideline update for the management of patients with chronic stable angina–summary article: a report of the American College of Cardiology/American Heart Association Task Force on Practice Guidelines (Committee on the Management of Patients With Chronic Stable Angina). Circulation 2003; 107:149–58
13. Hall FM. Language of the radiology report: primer for residents and wayward radiologists. AJR Am J Roentgenol 2000; 175:1239–42
14. Hamon M, Morello R, Riddell JW. Coronary arteries: diagnostic performance of 16- versus 64-section spiral CT compared with invasive coronary angiography–meta-analysis. Radiology 2007; 245:720–31
15. Herzog C, Ay M, Engelmann K, et al. Visualization techniques in multislice CT-coronary angiography of the heart. Correlations of axial, multiplanar, three-dimensional and virtual endoscopic imaging with the invasive diagnosis. Rofo 2001; 173:341–9
16. Hoe JW, Toh KH. A practical guide to reading CT coronary angiograms–how to avoid mistakes when assessing for coronary stenoses. Int J Cardiovasc Imaging 2007; 23:617–33
17. Hoffmann H, Dübel HP, Laube H, Hamm B, Dewey M. Triage of patients with suspected coronary artery disease using multislice computed tomography. Acad Radiol 2007; 14:901–9
18. Jacobs JE, Boxt LM, Desjardins B, Fishman EK, Larson PA, Schoepf J. ACR practice guideline for the performance and interpretation of cardiac computed tomography (CT). J Am Coll Radiol 2006; 3:677–85
19. Juergens KU, Fischbach R. Left ventricular function studied with MDCT. Eur Radiol 2006; 16:342–57
20. Kroft LJ, de Roos A, Geleijns J. Artifacts in ECG-synchronized MDCT coronary angiography. AJR Am J Roentgenol 2007; 189:581–91
21. Kushner DC, Lucey LL. Diagnostic radiology reporting and communication: the ACR guideline. J Am Coll Radiol 2005; 2:15–21
22. Leber AW, Becker A, Knez A, et al. Accuracy of 64-slice computed tomography to classify and quantify plaque volumes in the proximal coronary system: a comparative study using intravascular ultrasound. J Am Coll Cardiol 2006; 47:672–7
23. Libby P. Braunwald's Heart Disease: A Textbook of Cardiovascular Medicine: Saunders, An Imprint of Elsevier, 2007
24. MacMahon H, Austin JH, Gamsu G, et al. Guidelines for management of small pulmonary nodules detected on CT scans: a statement from the Fleischner Society. Radiology 2005; 237:395–400
25. Ryan TJ, Faxon DP, Gunnar RM, et al. Guidelines for percutaneous transluminal coronary angioplasty. a report of the American College of Cardiology/American Heart Association Task Force on Assessment of Diagnostic and Therapeutic Cardiovascular Procedures (Subcommittee on Percutaneous Transluminal Coronary Angioplasty). Circulation 1988; 78:486–502
26. Schnapauff D, Zimmermann E, Dewey M. Technical and clinical aspects of coronary computed tomography angiography. Semin Ultrasound CT MR 2008; 29:167–75
27. Smith SC, Jr, Dove JT, Jacobs AK, et al. ACC/AHA guidelines of percutaneous coronary interventions (revision of the 1993 PTCA guidelines)–executive summary. A report of the American College of Cardiology/American Heart Association Task Force on Practice Guidelines (committee to revise the 1993 guidelines for percutaneous transluminal coronary angioplasty). J Am Coll Cardiol 2001; 37:2215–39
28. Vogel-Claussen J, Pannu H, Spevak PJ, Fishman EK, Bluemke DA. Cardiac valve assessment with MR imaging and 64-section multidetector row CT. Radiographics 2006; 26:1769–84
29. Vogl TJ, Abolmaali ND, Diebold T, et al. Techniques for the detection of coronary atherosclerosis: multi-detector row CT coronary angiography. Radiology 2002; 223:212-20

The ACR practice guideline for the performance and interpretation of cardiac CT (Jacobs et al.) can be accessed at: http://www.acr.org/SecondaryMainMenuCategories/quality_safety/guidelines/dx/cardio/ct_cardiac.aspx

The ACR practice guideline for communication of diagnostic imaging findings (Kushner et al.) can be accessed at: http://www.acr.org/SecondaryMainMenuCategories/quality_safety/guidelines/dx/comm_diag_rad.aspx

Typical Clinical Examples

M. Dewey

10.1	Normal Coronary Arteries	129
10.2	Coronary Artery Plaques	132
10.3	Coronary Artery Stenoses	135
10.4	Coronary Artery Bypass Grafts	147
10.5	Coronary Artery Stents	156
10.6	Noncardiac Findings	164
10.7	Extracoronary Cardiac Findings	172

Abstract

This chapter summarizes the most common clinical examples of coronary CT angiography results.

10.1 Normal Coronary Arteries

The normal anatomy of different coronary artery distribution types as seen with multislice CT is presented in **Figs. 10.1–10.3**.

10.2 Coronary Artery Plaques

Coronary artery plaques of potentially different clinical importance are shown in **Figs. 10.4–10.7**.

10.3 Coronary Artery Stenoses

Significant coronary artery stenoses and occlusions and their variable appearance on coronary CT angiography, when compared with conventional invasive angiography, are shown in **Figs. 10.8–10.17**. See Chap. 11 for a summary of the diagnostic performance of coronary CT angiography in this application.

10.4 Coronary Artery Bypass Grafts

Arterial and venous coronary artery bypass grafts differ in diameter and are therefore more or less amenable to evaluation by CT. Examples are shown in **Figs. 10.18–10.26**. See Chap. 11 for a summary of the diagnostic performance of coronary CT angiography in this application.

10.5 Coronary Artery Stents

Evaluation of coronary artery stents is limited using today's technology, and if recommended at all, CT should only be used in patients with a single large-diameter (at least 3.5 mm) coronary stent. Typical results and issues involved in coronary CT stent imaging are shown in **Figs. 10.27–10.36**. See Chap. 11 for a summary of the diagnostic performance of coronary CT angiography in this application.

10.6 Noncardiac Findings

Noncardiac findings on coronary CT angiography are not uncommon and must be analyzed as meticulously as possible to ensure that important findings that might be responsible for a patient's symptoms are not missed and that unnecessary follow-up examinations are avoided. Common examples of noncardiac findings are provided in **Figs. 10.37–10.48**.

10.7 Extracoronary Cardiac Findings

Extracoronary cardiac findings are also quite common on coronary CT angiography and are important, in that they are often associated with the coronary findings and can be responsible for a patient's symptoms. Examples of typical extracoronary cardiac findings are provided in **Figs. 10.49–10.57**.

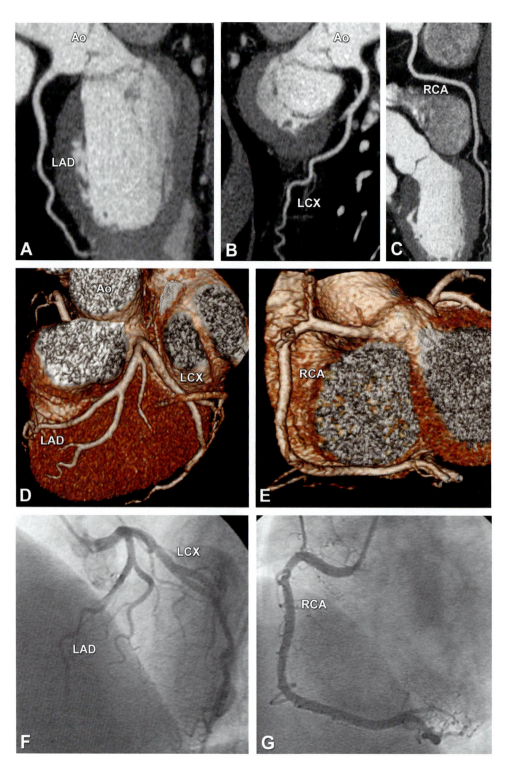

Fig. 10.1 Normal coronary arteries in a 56-year-old female patient presenting with nonanginal chest pain (see Chap. 5 for a description of angina types) and 0.2 mV (2 mm) ST segment depression in II, III, and aVF during stress testing (bicycle). **Panels A–C** show the curved multiplanar reformations along the left anterior descending (LAD), left circumflex (LCX), and right coronary (RCA) artery, respectively. Three-dimensional reconstructions of the left (**Panel D**) and right (**Panel E**) coronary artery are also unremarkable and demonstrate a codominant coronary distribution in this patient, which is found in 7–20% of all individuals. This distribution type is also seen on the corresponding conventional coronary angiograms of the left (**Panel F**) and right coronary artery (**Panel G**). Ruling out coronary artery disease in patients with low-to-intermediate pretest likelihood is the main application of coronary CT angiography. *Ao* aorta

10.1 • Normal Coronary Arteries

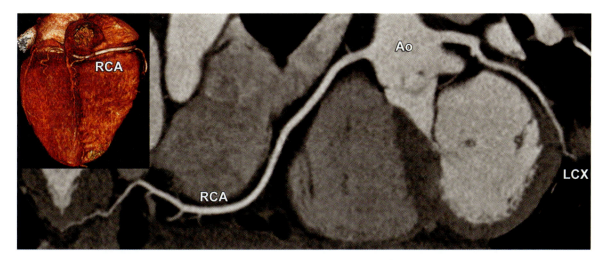

Fig. 10.2 Right coronary artery dominance, which is found in 60–85% of all individuals, as seen with CT using a curved multiplanar reformation along the right coronary (RCA) and left circumflex (LCX) coronary artery (inset shows the base of the heart with RCA dominance). *Ao* aorta

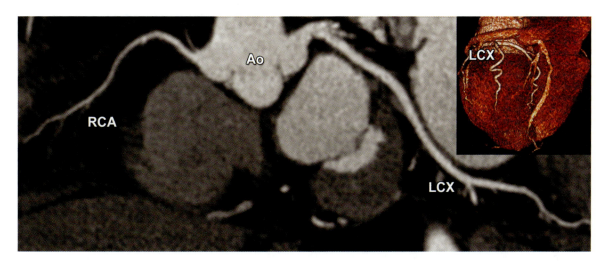

Fig. 10.3 Left coronary artery dominance, which is found in 7–20% of all individuals, as seen with CT using a curved multiplanar reformation along the right coronary (RCA) and left circumflex (LCX) coronary artery (inset shows the base of the heart with dominance of the LCX). *Ao* aorta

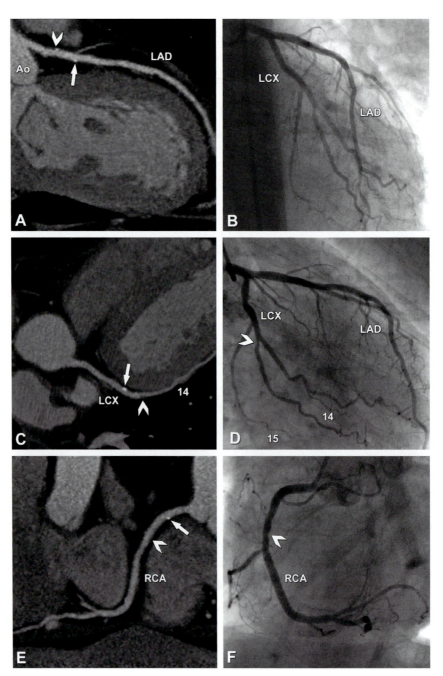

Fig. 10.4 No significant coronary artery stenoses, but small calcified plaques ("calcium spots") and noncalcified plaques in all coronaries in a 65-year-old male patient. The curved multiplanar reformation along the left anterior descending (LAD) coronary artery (**Panel A**) shows a calcium spot (*arrow*) and a mixed plaque (consisting of calcified and noncalcified components, *arrowhead*), which do not cause any indentation of the coronary lumen, as demonstrated by conventional coronary angiography (**Panel B**). There is another calcium spot (*arrow*) in the middle segment of the left circumflex coronary artery (LCX, **Panel C**) that does not cause any visible luminal narrowing on conventional angiography (**Panel D**), whereas a purely noncalcified plaque in the second obtuse marginal branch (*arrowhead*, segment 14) causes slight indentation of the coronary lumen (*arrowhead* in **Panel D**). The curved multiplanar reformation along the right coronary artery (RCA) shows the same findings (**Panel E**) with a calcium spot (*arrow*) not causing luminal narrowing, whereas the more distal noncalcified plaque in segment 2 (*arrowhead* in **Panel E**) is the cause of slight indentation (*arrowhead* in **Panel F**). *Ao* aorta; 15 = segment 15 (distal LCX)

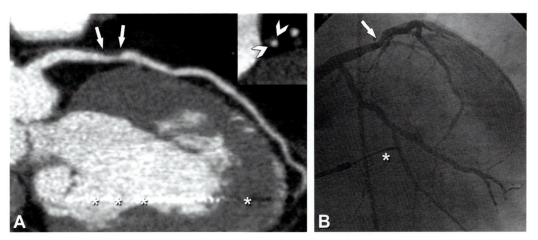

Fig. 10.5 Large noncalcified plaque in the proximal left anterior descending coronary artery (*arrows* in **Panel A**) of a 72-year-old male patient with typical angina pectoris (see Chap. 5 for a description of angina types). The plaque causes positive remodeling of the outer vessel wall (see inset in **Panel A**; *arrowheads* demarcate the boundaries of this plaque). The so-called remodeling index is defined as the ratio of the vessel area at the plaque site (including plaque and lumen area) to the mean of the vessel area at the reference site proximal and distal to the plaque. Positive remodeling, as in this case, is present if the index is >1.05 and indicates an increased risk for unstable presentation of patients. However, the value of potential clinical consequences (e.g., initiation or increase in statin therapy) in patients with noncalcified plaques without significant luminal narrowing but positive remodeling has not been established. This plaque (*arrow*) caused a 35% diameter stenosis, as measured with quantitative analysis of coronary angiography (**Panel B**). Note the artifacts in CT (*asterisks* in **Panel A**) arising from the cardiac pacemaker lead (*asterisk* in **Panel B**)

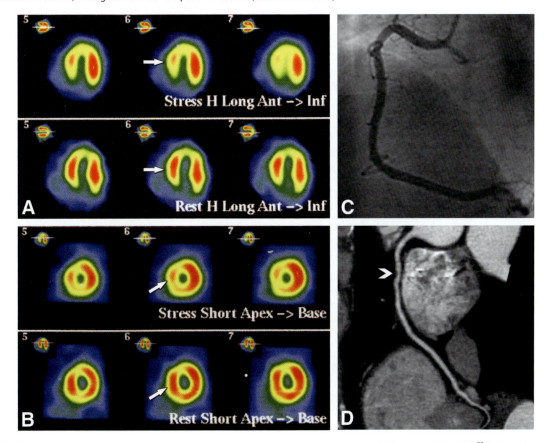

Fig. 10.6 Example of a false-positive single-photon emission computed tomography (SPECT) examination with ^{99m}Tc in a 68-year-old male patient with reduced septal and inferior stress perfusion (*arrows* in **Panels A** and **B**). These findings were suggestive of a significant stenosis in the right coronary artery. The right coronary artery, however, was normal and without signs of significant stenosis on conventional coronary angiography (**Panel C**) or coronary CT angiography (curved multiplanar reformation, **Panel D**). However, there was a noncalcified coronary plaque in the midsegment of the right coronary artery on CT (*arrowhead* in **Panel D**) that was not visible on conventional angiography and might have been responsible for the SPECT findings

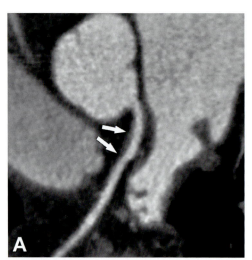
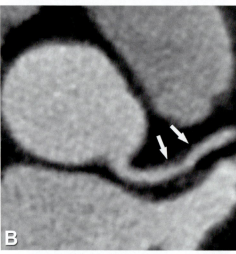
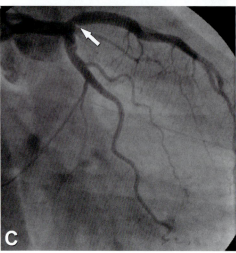

Fig. 10.7 Large noncalcified plaque (*arrows* in **Panels A** and **B**) in the proximal left anterior descending coronary artery in a 58-year-old female patient with typical angina pectoris. The CT results are illustrated using a curved multiplanar reformation (**Panel A**) and maximum-intensity projection (**Panel B**). This plaque also results in positive remodeling (remodeling index of >1.05), but the indentation of the coronary artery lumen (from below, *arrow* in **Panel C**) is not significant (30% diameter stenosis on quantitative analysis)

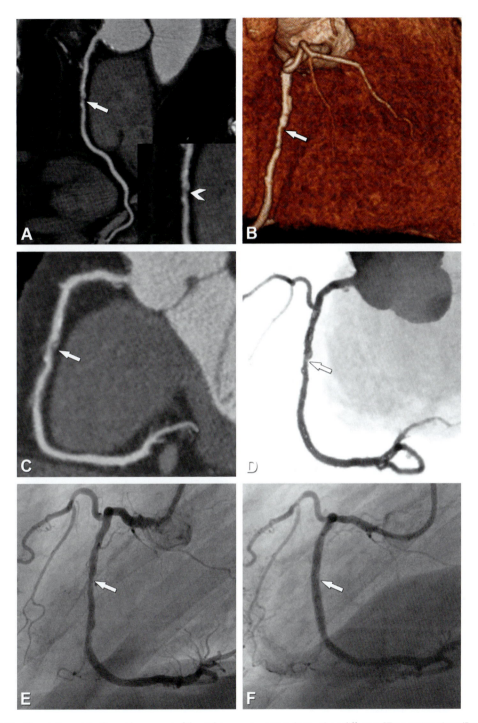

Fig. 10.8 Significant stenosis in the mid-segment of the right coronary artery (*arrows*) on different CT reconstructions (**Panels A–D**) in a 62-year-old male patient with typical angina pectoris but unremarkable exercise ECG. Reconstructions of CT include curved multiplanar reformation (**Panel A**, inset shows the stenosis [*arrowhead*] in a magnified view), volume-rendered three-dimensional reconstruction (**Panel B**), thin-slab maximum-intensity projection curved along the vessel path (so-called CATH view, **Panel C**), and angiographic emulation (**Panel D**). There was good correlation with the findings on subsequently performed conventional coronary angiography (*arrow* in **Panel E**). During the same invasive angiographic examination, this lesion was treated percutaneously with stent placement, with no residual stenosis (*arrow* in **Panel F**)

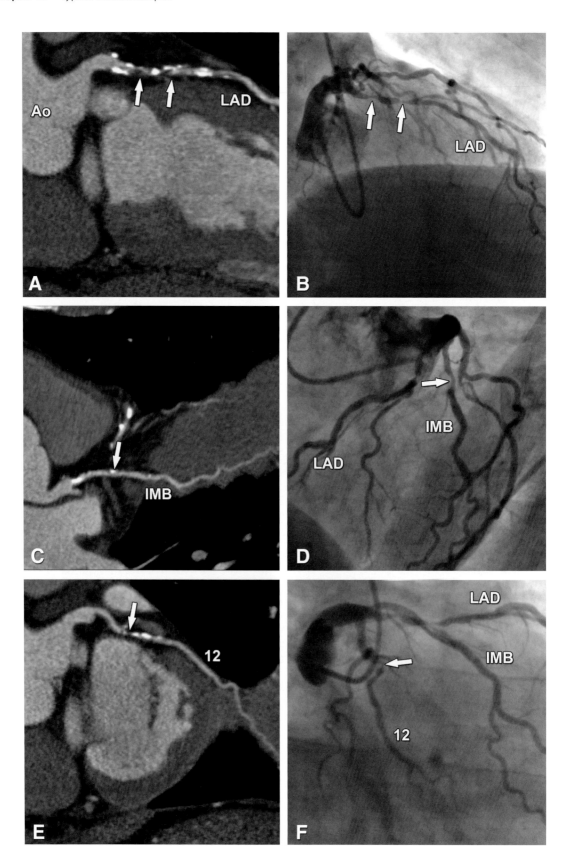

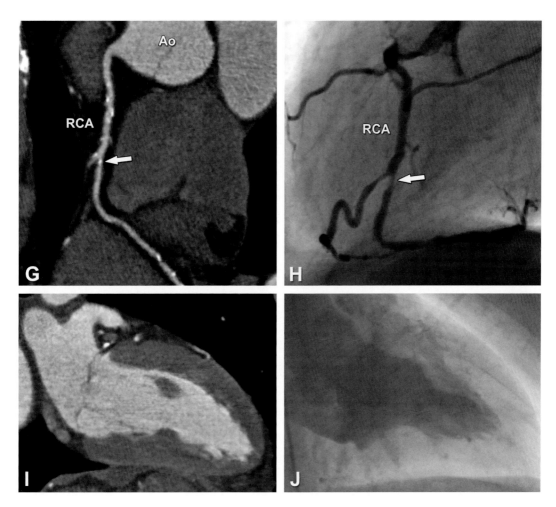

Fig. 10.9 Significant stenoses (*arrows*) in the four main coronary vessels in a 63-year-old male patient with typical angina pectoris and 0.2 mV (2 mm) ST segment depression on exercise ECG in II, III, and aVF indicating posterior ischemia. Coronary CT results are shown as curved multiplanar reformations along the vessels (left column) and are directly compared with conventional coronary angiography (right column, stenosis degrees obtained with quantitative analysis). There are two 80% diameter stenoses (*arrows*) in the proximal and mid-segment of the left anterior descending coronary artery (LAD, **Panels A** and **B**). These result mainly from noncalcified plaques in these two segments (**Panel A**). However, there are also severely calcified plaques that do not result in significant diameter reductions. An intermediate branch (IMB) is present in this patient and has a 65% diameter stenosis resulting from a calcified plaque (**Panels C** and **D**) There is another short significant coronary stenosis resulting from a noncalcified plaque in the first obtuse marginal branch (segment 12, **Panels E** and **F**), with a diameter stenosis on conventional coronary angiography of 75% that was clearly overestimated on CT (90–95%, **Panel E**). In contrast, the 80% diameter stenosis of the mid-right coronary artery (RCA, **Panel H**), as determined by quantitative coronary angiography, was underestimated by CT as only 65% (**Panel G**). Global left ventricular ejection fraction was 53% on CT (end-systolic two-chamber view, **Panel I**) and 50% on cineventriculography (end-systolic right anterior oblique view, **Panel J**). Thus, according to guidelines (Chap. 9) percutaneous stenting, rather than coronary bypass grafting, was initiated (beginning with the stenosis in the RCA responsible for the ischemic findings on exercise testing). *Ao* aorta

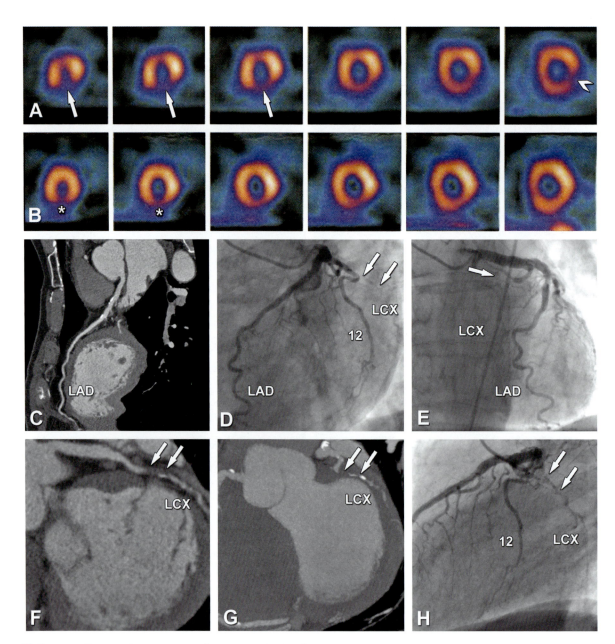

Fig. 10.10 Two-vessel coronary artery disease correctly identified on single-photon emission computed tomography (SPECT) myocardial perfusion imaging (**Panels A** and **B**) and coronary CT angiography (**Panels C, F, G, I,** and **J**) in a 65-year-old male patient with a one-month history of atypical angina pectoris. SPECT shows ischemia in the apical and mid-inferior segments (*arrows* in **Panel A**, short-axis views) that correlates with less markedly reduced perfusion in the same segments at rest (*asterisks* in **Panel B**). In addition, SPECT shows ischemia in the basal inferolateral segment (*arrowhead* in **Panel A**). Coronary CT angiography shows no significant stenosis in the left anterior descending coronary artery, but only calcified plaques (LAD, **Panel C**). This finding is in agreement with conventional angiography (**Panels D** and **E**). However, there is a 10-mm-long occlusion of the mid-left circumflex coronary artery (LCX) caused by a mainly noncalcified plaque, as seen with CT (*arrows* in **Panels F** and **G**). **Panel F** is a curved multiplanar reformation along the vessel path, and **Panel G** is a maximum-intensity projection. Conventional coronary angiography confirms the presence of the occlusion but fails to exactly determine the length of the occlusion (*arrows* in **Panels D, E,** and **H**), while it nicely demonstrates the presence of right-to-left collaterals bridging the LCX occlusion (*asterisks* in **Panel K**)

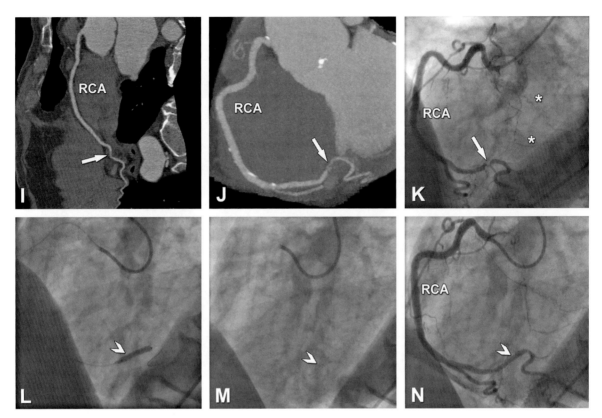

Fig. 10.10 (continued) Both CT (**Panels I** and **J**) and conventional angiography (**Panel K**) depict a rather short significant 80% diameter stenosis (*arrow*) at the crux cordis in the right coronary artery (RCA). Since the occlusion was considered to be a long-standing process, the recent onset of symptoms was most likely due to the reduction in collateral flow to the LCX because of the RCA stenosis. Thus, the RCA stenosis was stented (*arrowheads*) in the same angiographic session, with good technical success (**Panels L–N**)

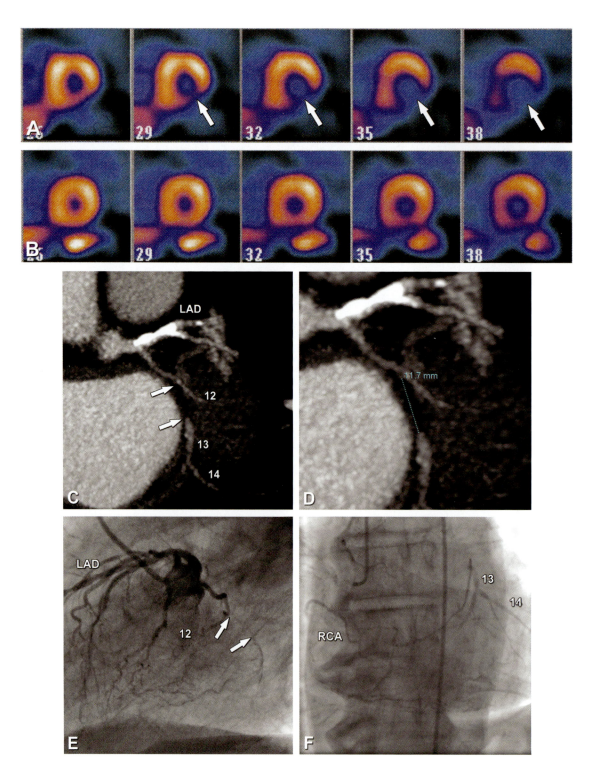

Fig. 10.11 Occlusion of the left circumflex coronary artery (LCX) in a 72-year-old male patient with atypical angina pectoris. There is basal and mid-cavity inferolateral and posterior ischemia (*arrows*) on single-photon emission computed tomography (SPECT) myocardial perfusion imaging (**Panel A**, stress exam). There was no perfusion deficit during the examination of SPECT at rest (**Panel B**). Coronary CT angiography shows a 12 mm-long occlusion (*arrows* and measurement) of the mid-LCX (segment 13) as a result of a noncalcified plaque just distal to the branching of a small obtuse marginal artery (segment 12, **Panels C** and **D**, maximum-intensity projections). Conventional coronary angiography nicely shows the occlusion (*arrows* in **Panel E**) and demonstrates right-to-left collaterals, with filling of the middle and distal left circumflex coronary segments (**Panel F**). Despite the purely noncalcified occlusion, percutaneous revascularization failed, most likely because of the location at a branching obtuse marginal artery. Note that during this angiographic session, the left anterior descending coronary artery (LAD) was successfully revascularized. *RCA* right coronary artery

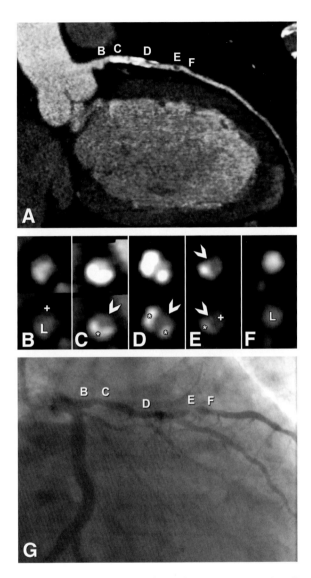

Fig. 10.12 Diffuse atherosclerotic changes in the left anterior descending coronary artery in a 63-year-old male patient with typical angina pectoris (curved multiplanar reformation of CT in **Panel A**). For correlation, cross-sections orthogonal to the curved multiplanar reformation along the vessel obtained by CT (**Panels B–F**) and conventional coronary angiography (**Panel G**) are provided. The letters from B to F indicate matching sites on CT (**Panel A**) and conventional angiography (**Panel G**). The corresponding cross-sections are provided in **Panels B–F** using standard coronary artery settings (*top row*) and bone-window-like settings (*bottom row*). Interestingly, despite the diffuse changes, there is only one significant luminal narrowing (90% diameter stenosis) of the coronary artery (*arrowhead* in **Panel E**), which is caused by a noncalcified plaque (*plus* in **Panel E**) and calcified plaque (*asterisk* in **Panel E**). Note that the residual lumen at the site of this plaque is better appreciated using the standard coronary artery window-level settings (*arrowhead* in the *upper row* in **Panel E**). In contrast, the stenosis diameter at the sites of highly calcified coronary artery plaques (*asterisks* in the *bottom row* in **Panels C** and **D**) is more easily evaluated using bone-window settings (*arrowheads* in the *bottom row* in **Panels C** and **D**). The proximal vessel segments (B in **Panel G**) and distal vessel segments (F in **Panel G**) appear very similar on conventional coronary angiography (**Panel G**). However, CT shows a relevant difference, with a large noncalcified plaque (*plus* in **Panel B**) proximally without luminal narrowing (*L* in **Panel B**), but no such atherosclerotic changes in the distal vessel segment (**Panel F**). This difference underscores the underestimation of the extent of atherosclerosis with conventional coronary angiography, which is well known from necropsy and intravascular ultrasound studies

Chapter 10 · Typical Clinical Examples

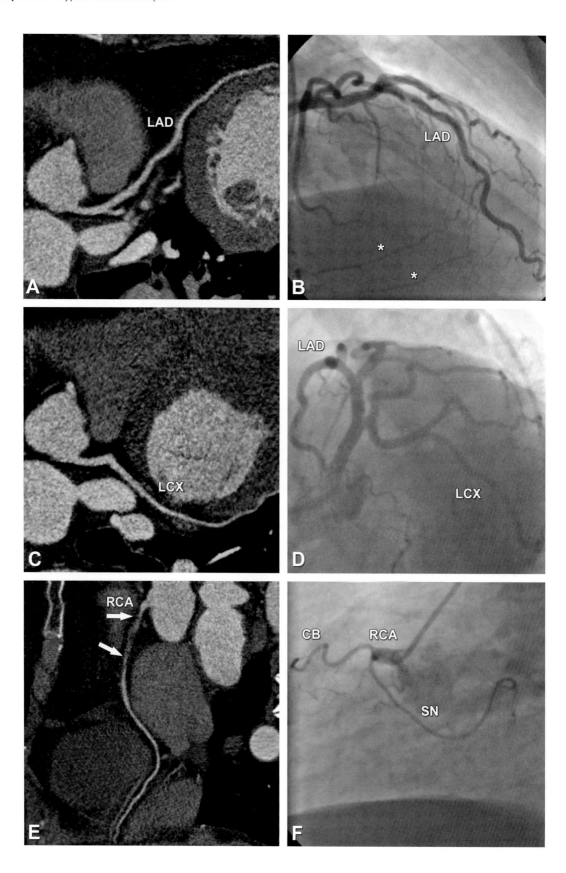

Fig. 10.13 Occlusion of the right coronary artery (RCA) in a 53-year-old male patient with rather atypical presentation (see Chap. 5 for a description of angina types) and 0.05 mV (0.5 mm) ST segment depression during stress testing in II, III, and aVF indicating posterior ischemia. There are no significant stenoses in the left anterior descending (LAD in **Panels A** and **B**) and left circumflex coronary artery (LCX in **Panels C** and **D**) as seen with coronary CT (curved multiplanar reformations in **Panels A** and **C**) and conventional coronary angiography (**Panels B** and **D**). The occlusion in the proximal and middle segments of the RCA extends over a length of 4 cm and is not calcified (*arrows* in **Panel E**). Because of the short distance from the ostium of the RCA to the beginning of the occlusion (0.5 cm, **Panel F**), percutaneous revascularization was unsuccessful. Note that CT is superior to invasive angiography in identifying the exact length of the occlusion (*arrows* in **Panel E**). Coronary bypass surgery was not considered as an option in this patient because there was good left-to-right collateralization of the occlusion (*asterisks* in **Panel B**), and the patient had only mild symptoms. However, medical therapy was optimized. *CB* conus branch; *SN* sinus node artery

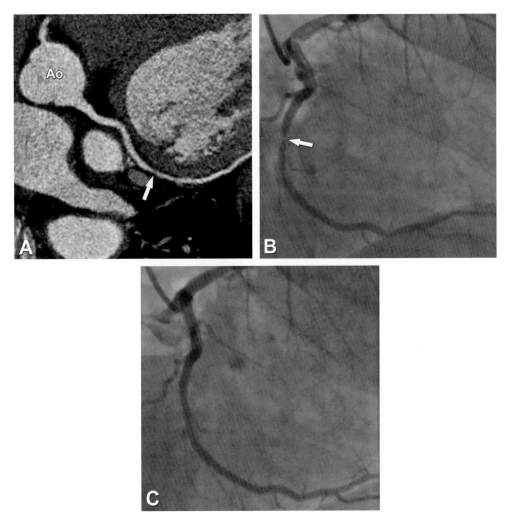

Fig. 10.14 Significant stenosis of the left circumflex coronary artery (*arrows*) in a 76-year-old male patient with typical angina pectoris, as seen with CT (**Panel A**) and conventional coronary angiography (**Panel B**). Measurement of the percent diameter stenosis resulted in values of 70% for CT and 75% for conventional angiography (with quantitative analysis). The stenosis was caused by a noncalcified plaque (*arrow* in **Panel A**). The outcome of percutaneous coronary intervention is shown in **Panel C**

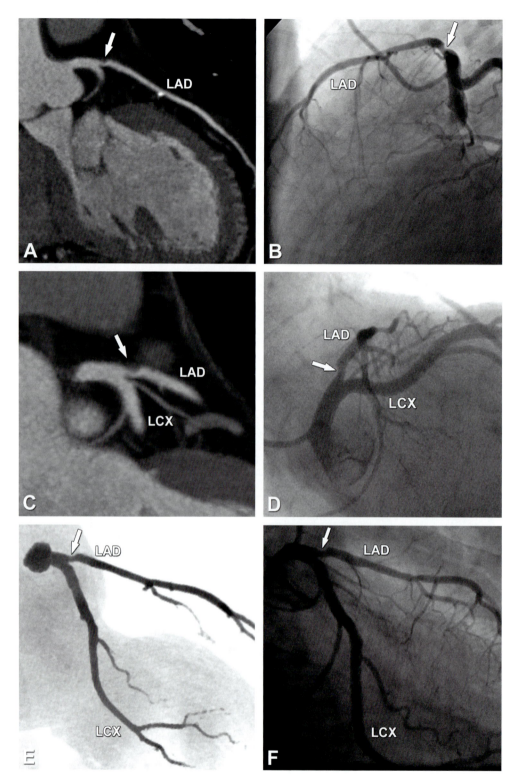

Fig. 10.15 Borderline stenosis (*arrows*) of the proximal left anterior descending coronary artery (LAD) in a 62-year-old male patient with typical angina pectoris, as seen with CT (*left column*) and conventional angiography (*right column*). Results of coronary CT angiography are shown as a curved multiplanar reformation (**Panel A**), thin-slab maximum-intensity projection (**Panel C**), and angiographic emulation (**Panel E**). There is good correlation with the corresponding invasive angiogram projections (**Panels B**, **D**, and **F**). Both CT and quantitative conventional coronary angiography estimated a percent diameter stenosis of 50%. Because there were no signs of ischemia on exercise ECG, no revascularization was attempted. With optimized medical management, the patient's angina pectoris resolved. Note that there is a small calcified plaque in the mid-LAD (**Panel A**). *LCX* left circumflex coronary artery

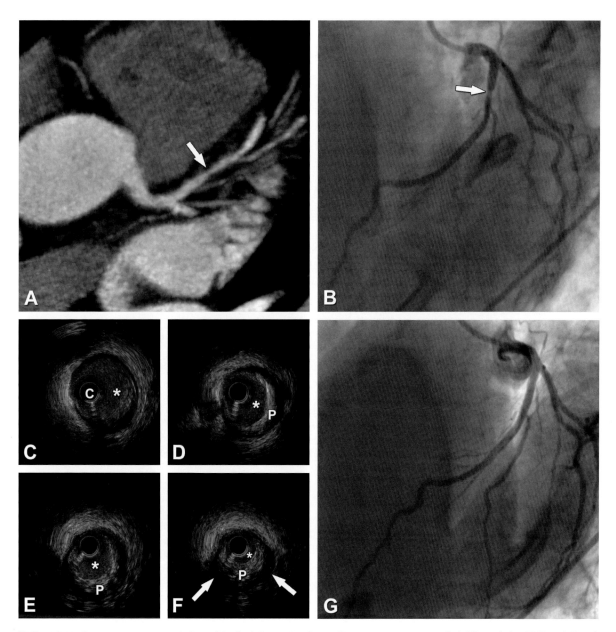

Fig. 10.16 Coronary artery stenosis (*arrow*) in the left anterior descending coronary artery, graded differently by CT (**Panel A**) and invasive angiography (**Panel B**) in a 62-year-old female patient with typical angina pectoris and ST segment depression of 0.15 mV (1.5 mm) in V4–6 during stress testing (bicycle) indicating anterior ischemia. CT shows a short 70% diameter stenosis caused by a noncalcified plaque in the proximal vessel segment with positive remodeling (**Panel A**, maximum-intensity projection), whereas quantitative analysis of conventional angiography shows only a 40% diameter reduction. Because of worsening angina pectoris and the coronary CT findings, repeat angiography, including intravascular ultrasound (**Panels C–F**), was performed 6 months later. Intravascular ultrasound (cross-sections), located from proximal LAD to the stenosis, confirmed the presence of the plaque (*P* in **Panels D–F**) that caused a short 70% diameter stenosis (*arrows* in **Panel F**) of the lumen (*asterisk* in **Panels C–F**). On the basis of these findings, percutaneous coronary intervention was performed (**Panel G**). *C* intravascular ultrasound catheter

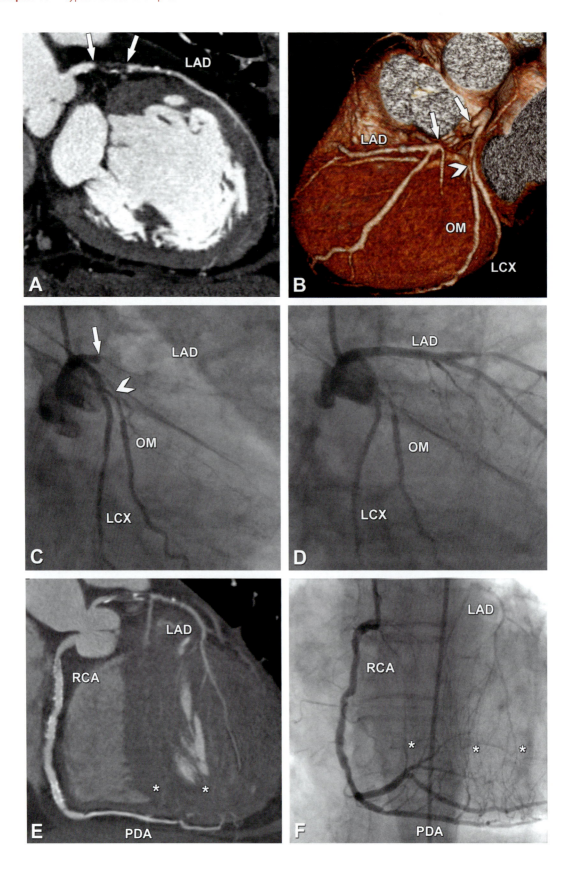

10.4 · Coronary Artery Bypass Grafts

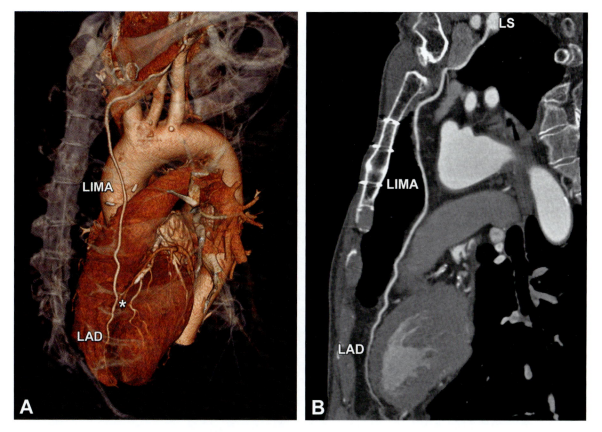

◘ **Fig. 10.18** Normal left internal mammary artery (LIMA) coronary bypass graft to the left anterior descending coronary artery (LAD). The CT data are shown in a three-dimensional volume-rendered reconstruction (left anterosuperior view, **Panel A**), with the distal anastomosis indicated by an *asterisk*. The curved multiplanar reformation along the arterial graft (including its origin from the left subclavian artery, LS) is shown in **Panel B**

◘ **Fig. 10.17** Occlusion of the proximal left anterior descending coronary artery (LAD) in a 78-year-old female patient with a 2-week history of typical angina pectoris (*arrows* in **Panels A–C**). A curved multiplanar reformation of CT is shown in **Panel A**, while **Panel B** is a volume-rendered three-dimensional reconstruction. There is an excellent correlation with conventional coronary angiography, and the length (1.5 cm) of the occlusion, which was mainly caused by a noncalcified plaque, is better seen with CT (*arrows* in **Panel A**). Percutaneous coronary intervention was performed during the same angiographic session, and good revascularization was achieved (compare **Panel D** with **Panel C**). There was also a significant stenosis (*arrowhead* in **Panels B** and **C**) of the obtuse marginal artery (OM) of the left circumflex coronary artery (LCX). The LAD occlusion was collateralized via septal branches (*asterisks* in **Panels E** and **F**) arising from the posterior descending coronary artery (PDA). **Panel E** is a CATH view (curved thin-slab maximum-intensity projection) of coronary CT angiography along the right coronary artery (RCA). This CT reconstruction is superior in that it depicts both the RCA with the collaterals (*asterisks*) and the LAD (with the occlusion) in a single image

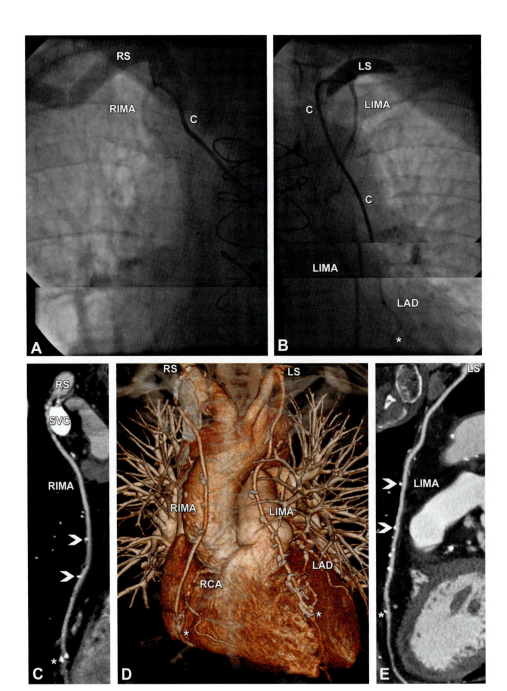

Fig. 10.19 Advantages of coronary CT angiography in depicting coronary bypasses. Example of patent coronary arterial bypass grafts in a 68-year-old male patient with typical angina pectoris who underwent bypass grafting 7 years earlier. Conventional coronary angiography failed to demonstrate patency of the graft because it was not possible to selectively insert the catheter into the right internal mammary artery (RIMA, **Panel A**). *C* indicates the position of the catheter. The left internal mammary artery (LIMA) coronary bypass to the left anterior descending coronary artery (LAD) including the distal anastomosis (*asterisk*) was normal on conventional angiography (**Panel B**). CT was initiated, and in contrast to the conventional angiograms, it was able to demonstrate a normal RIMA graft to the right coronary artery (RCA) on both a curved multiplanar reformation (**Panel C**) and a three-dimensional volume-rendered reconstruction (*anterior view*, **Panel D**). Coronary CT angiography also confirmed the patency of the LIMA to the LAD (**Panels D** and **E**). Note the metallic surgical clips along the arterial bypass grafts (*arrowheads* in **Panels C** and **E**) and the distal anastomoses (*asterisk* in **Panels C** and **E**). Very dense contrast material is still present in the superior vena cava (SVC) because the injection was performed via a right cubital vein. Deviating from the standard procedure of contrast injection into the right arm veins and using left-sided injection instead might have been preferable in this patient. This way, LIMA assessment might have been limited, but CT was primarily performed because conventional angiography was nondiagnostic with regard to the RIMA graft. *C* catheter; *LS* left subclavian artery; *RS* right subclavian artery

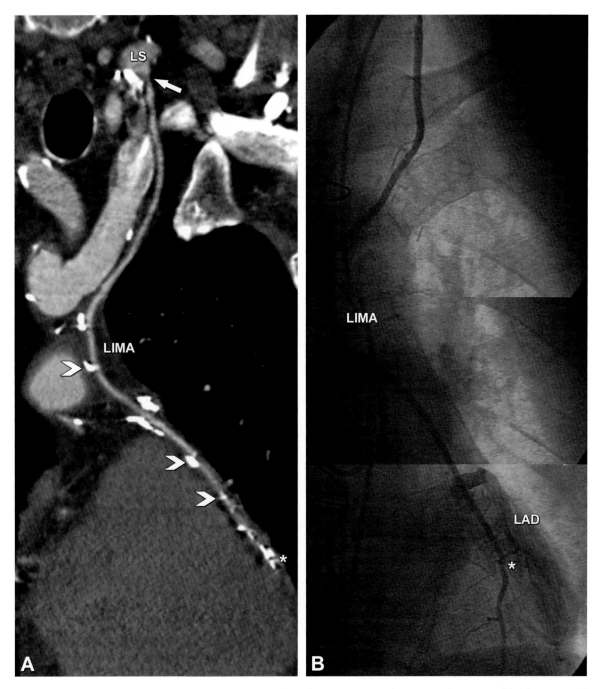

Fig. 10.20 Advantages of conventional coronary angiography in depicting coronary bypasses. In this 74-year-old male patient with atypical angina pectoris who underwent left internal mammary artery (LIMA) coronary bypass grafting to the left anterior descending coronary artery (LAD) 4 years ago, CT was unable to rule out significant stenoses because of artifacts arising from nearby dense contrast material in the veins (*arrow*) and surgical clips (*arrowheads* in **Panel A**, curved multiplanar reformation). Also, the distal anastomosis (*asterisk*) could not be reliably assessed with CT (**Panel A**). In contrast, subsequently performed conventional angiography shows a patent LIMA to LAD (**Panel B**). Newer surgical clips have a lower metal content and therefore tend to produce fewer artifacts on coronary CT

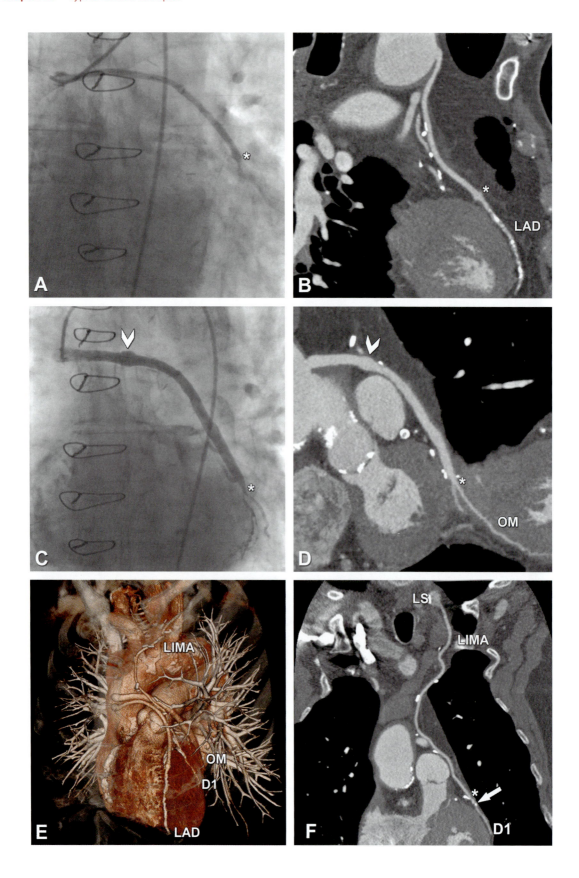

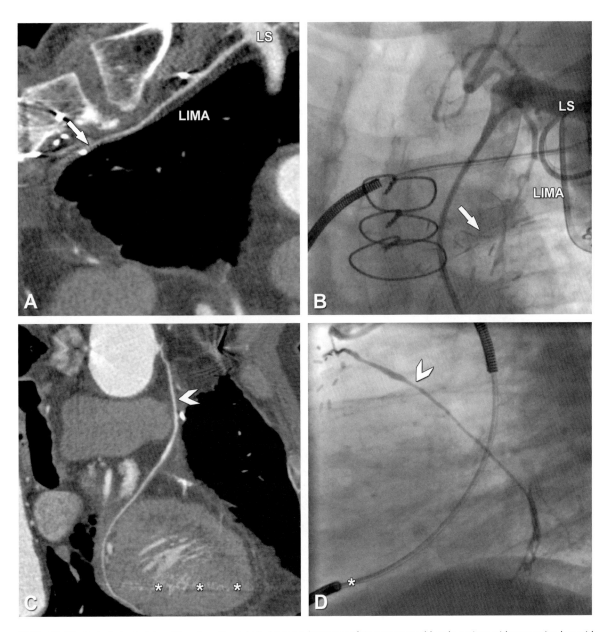

Fig. 10.22 Occluded arterial and functionally occluded venous bypass graft in a 66-year-old male patient without angina but with severe dyspnea. Curved multiplanar reformation along the left internal mammary artery (LIMA) shows occlusion about 5–6 cm from the origin (*arrow* in **Panel A**). There is good agreement with the findings from conventional angiography (**Panel B**). The venous bypass graft to the obtuse marginal artery has a very small diameter of only 1 mm (*arrowhead*) and is functionally occluded, as seen on CT (**Panel C**, curved multiplanar reformation) and conventional angiography (**Panel D**). Note that the patient has an implanted cardiac defibrillator (*asterisk* in **Panel D**), which leads to minor artifacts on CT (*asterisks* in **Panel C**). *LS* left subclavian artery

Fig. 10.21 Normal coronary arterial and venous bypass grafts in a 79-year-old male patient. There is good correlation of conventional angiography (**Panels A** and **C**) and CT (**Panels B** and **D**) in the evaluation of the venous bypass grafts to the left anterior descending coronary artery (LAD, **Panels A** and **B**) and the obtuse marginal artery (OM, **Panels C** and **D**). There is focal dilatation of the venous graft to the OM due to a venous valve (*arrowhead* in **Panels C** and **D**), while the distal anastomoses (*asterisk*) are unremarkable (**Panels A–D**). However, conventional angiography was unsuccessful in aiding the selective insertion of a catheter into the left internal mammary artery (LIMA). Thus, CT was initiated and was able to visualize this graft to the first diagonal branch (D1). Three-dimensional and curved multiplanar reformations of the LIMA graft are shown in **Panels E** and **F**, respectively. The distal anastomosis of this graft was normal (*asterisk* in **Panel F**), but there was a significant stenosis of the D1 (*arrow* in **Panel F**), which was also seen on conventional coronary angiography. *LS* left subclavian artery

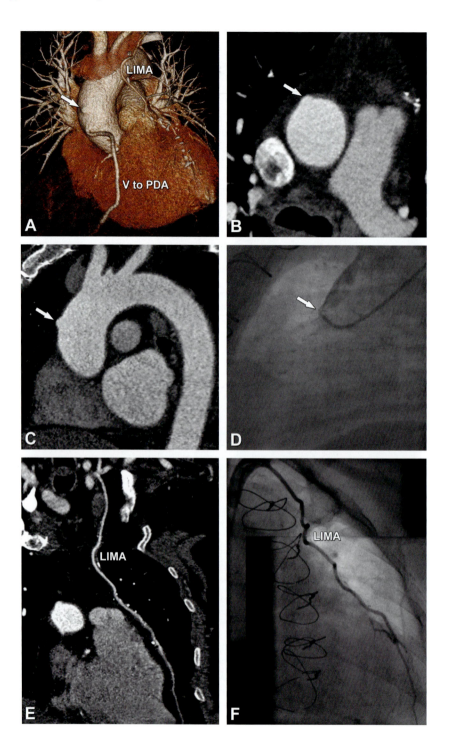

Fig. 10.23 Comprehensive assessment of coronary bypass grafts and native coronary arteries in a 64-year-old female patient with atypical angina pectoris. There is ostial occlusion of the venous bypass graft, which passed to the left circumflex coronary artery, as can be seen in the three-dimensional reconstruction of CT (*arrow* in **Panel A**). In axial source images and a sagittal reconstruction of CT, the occlusion (*arrow*) looks like a small outpouching of the lumen (**Panels B** and **C**). Conventional angiography confirmed the occlusion (*arrow* in **Panel D**). The left internal mammary artery (LIMA) is patent to the left anterior descending coronary artery (**Panels E** and **F**), but CT detected significant stenosis at the distal anastomosis (*arrows*) of the venous bypass graft to the posterior descending coronary artery (V to PDA, **Panel G**)

10.4 · Coronary Artery Bypass Grafts

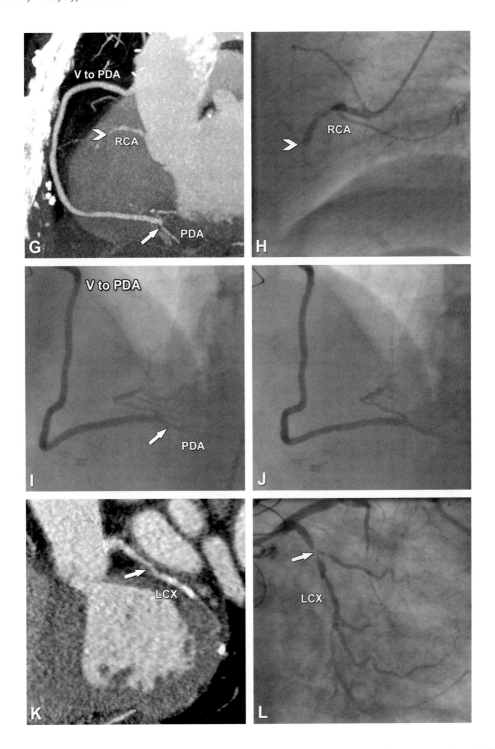

Fig. 10.23 (continued) **Panel G** is a maximum-intensity projection demonstrating the stenosis at the anastomosis to the PDA (*arrow*). The right coronary artery (RCA) is occluded at the junction of segments 1 and 2 (*arrowhead* in **Panel G**). Both the occlusion of the RCA (*arrowhead* in **Panel H**) and the stenosis at the distal anastomosis of the venous bypass graft to the posterior descending coronary artery (*arrow* in **Panel I**) were confirmed by subsequently performed conventional angiography. During the same angiographic session, percutaneous coronary stenting of the stenosis of the distal anastomosis was performed (**Panel J**). CT also found a significant stenosis (*arrow*) of the left circumflex coronary artery (LCX, **Panel K**), which was confirmed by conventional angiography (*arrow* in **Panel L**) and was also treated interventionally

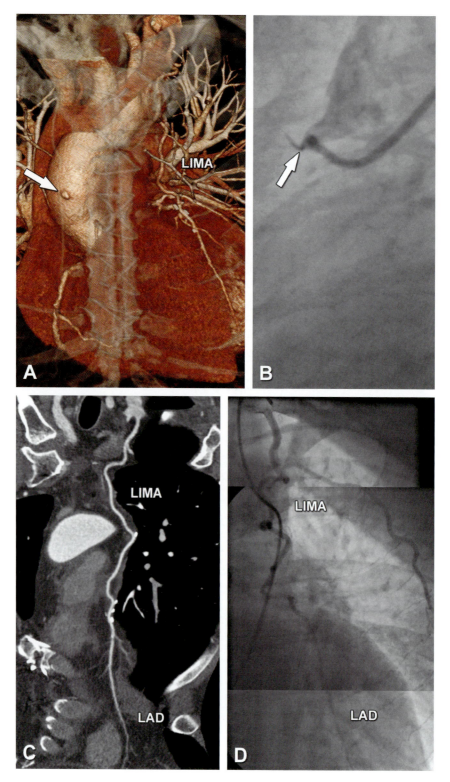

Fig. 10.24 Occluded venous bypass graft and patent left internal mammary artery (LIMA) in a 64-year-old male patient with atypical angina. Ostial occlusion of the venous bypass graft (*arrow*) that supplies the left circumflex coronary artery (**Panel A**). **Panel A** is a three-dimensional reconstruction (anterior view). This finding was confirmed by conventional coronary angiography (lateral projection, *arrow* in **Panel B**). The LIMA to the left anterior descending coronary artery (LAD) was unremarkable on both CT (curved multiplanar reformation, **Panel C**) and conventional angiography (**Panel D**)

10.4 · Coronary Artery Bypass Grafts

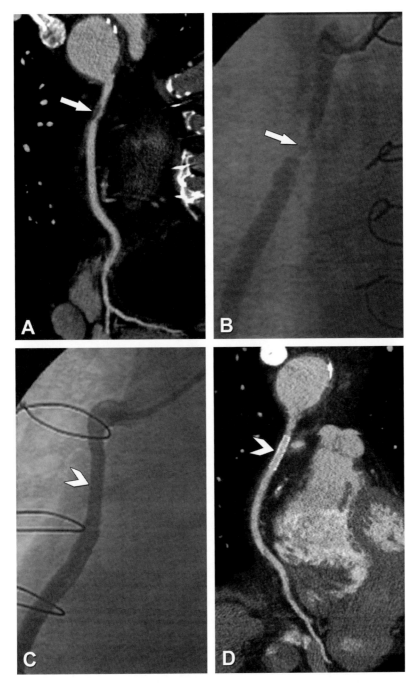

Fig. 10.25 Stenosis of a venous coronary bypass graft in a 69-year-old male patient with typical angina pectoris. Curved multiplanar reformation of CT shows a noncalcified plaque (*arrow*) in the proximal portion of a venous bypass graft to the right coronary artery, resulting in 80% diameter stenosis (**Panel A**) as measured with digital calipers on orthogonal cross-sections. Subsequently performed conventional angiography confirmed this finding (*arrow* in **Panel B**), and during the same angiographic session, percutaneous intervention with a 4.0-mm stent was performed (*arrowhead* in **Panel C**). Follow-up CT demonstrated a patent stent without significant in-stent restenosis (*arrowhead* in **Panel D**)

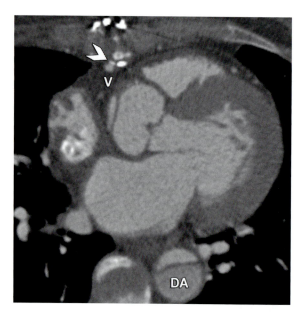

Fig. 10.26 Prior to reoperative cardiac surgery, CT can identify important findings. In this patient, a sternal wire (*arrowhead*) is located near a venous bypass graft (V). Also, the distance from the sternum to bypasses can be easily measured using CT before reoperation. In this case, there was also a dissection of the descending aorta (DA)

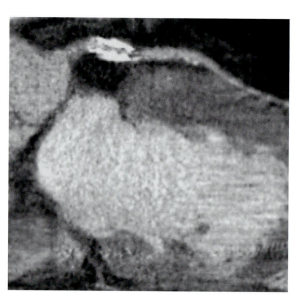

Fig. 10.28 Nondiagnostic coronary artery stent in the proximal left anterior descending coronary artery (curved multiplanar reformation) in a 64-year-old male patient with nonanginal chest pain. Despite the large diameter of the stent (4.0 mm), the lumen was not evaluable because of motion and beam-hardening artifacts. Interestingly, stents as large as this one are implanted in only about a fifth of all cases, and the vast majority of patients receive coronary stents of 2.5 or 3.0 mm in diameter, which can be reliably evaluated by CT in only 50% of the time (Chap. 11)

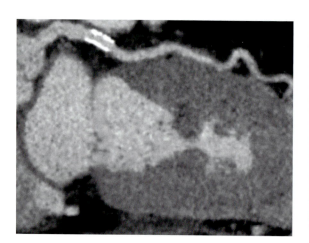

Fig. 10.27 Patent coronary artery stent (3.5-mm diameter) with good runoff in the proximal left anterior descending coronary artery (curved multiplanar reformation) in a 58-year-old female patient presenting with typical angina pectoris

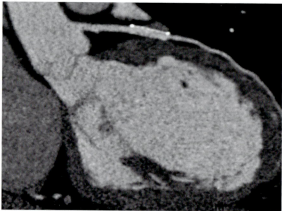

Fig. 10.29 Patent coronary artery stent (3.0-mm diameter) in the proximal left anterior descending coronary artery (curved multiplanar reformation) in a 41-year-old male patient who was asymptomatic but at high risk (history of acute anterior myocardial infarction and stenting at the age of 36). Note the irregular vessel wall immediately distal from the stent that did not result in significant stenosis

10.5 · Coronary Artery Stents

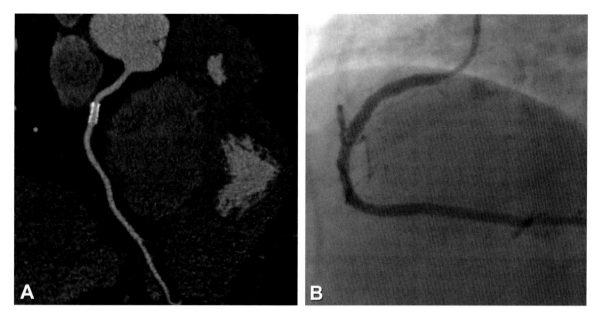

Fig. 10.30 Patent coronary artery stent (4.0 mm diameter) in the mid-right coronary artery without significant restenosis (curved multiplanar reformation, **Panel A**) in a 64-year-old male patient presenting with typical angina pectoris. There is good agreement in this large-diameter stent with conventional coronary angiography (**Panel B**)

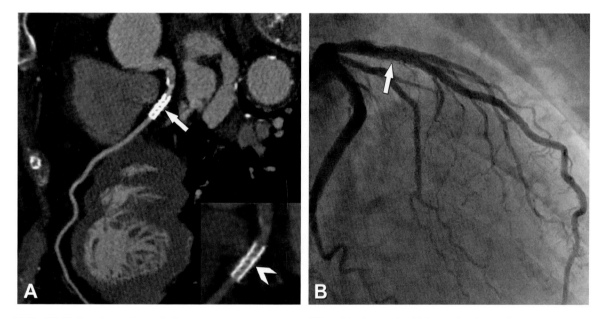

Fig. 10.31 Nondiagnostic small-diameter coronary artery stent (2.5 mm) in the proximal left anterior descending coronary artery (*arrow* in **Panel A**, curved multiplanar reformation) in an 80-year-old female patient presenting with typical angina pectoris. The runoff seems excellent but this is not a reliable sign on its own in excluding significant in-stent restenosis; enhancement may as well be caused by collateral flow that can be overlooked in nondynamic CT imaging. Even stent kernel reconstructions (inset in **Panel A**, *arrowhead*, curved multiplanar reformation) did not allow reliable exclusion of significant in-stent restenosis in this case. Conventional coronary angiography (**Panel B**) showed some neointimal proliferation (*arrow*) but no significant in-stent restenosis

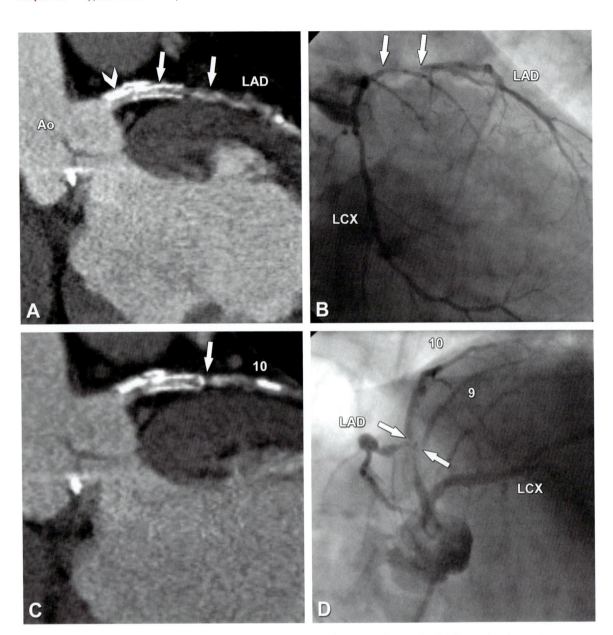

Fig. 10.32 Significant restenosis of a 3.0 mm diameter bare-metal stent in the proximal left anterior descending coronary artery (LAD) in a 63-year-old male with typical angina pectoris. Coronary CT angiography suggested occlusion of this stent (*arrows* in **Panel A**, curved multiplanar reformation). There was also a large calcified plaque in the left main coronary artery that did not cause significant luminal narrowing (*asterisk* in **Panel A**). In contrast, quantitative analysis of conventional coronary angiography demonstrated that there was no occlusion, but 90% in-stent restenosis had occurred (*arrows* in **Panel B**). Because of its lower spatial resolution, CT is often unable to differentiate high-grade stenosis from occlusion. Because of the location of the stent at the branchings of the first (9) and second (10) diagonal branches, a complex situation involving a trifurcation stenosis was present (*arrows* in **Panels C** and **D**). The left circumflex coronary artery (LCX) had no significant stenosis (**Panel D**)

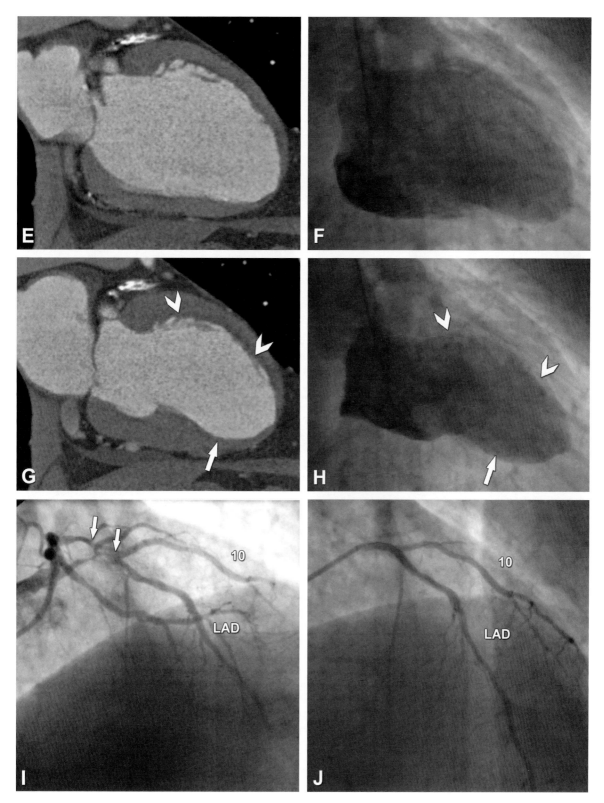

Fig. 10.32 (continued) There was extensive akinesia of the apical inferior segment (*arrow*) and hypokinesia of the midventricular and apical anterior segments (*arrowheads*) in the two-chamber view on CT (**Panels E** and **G**) and in the right anterior oblique projection by cineventriculography (**Panels F** and **H**, with **Panels E** and **F** representing end-diastole and **Panels G** and **H** representing end-systole). During the same angiographic session, successful complex percutaneous intervention of the LAD and the second diagonal branch (10) was performed (**Panels I–J**). *Ao* aorta

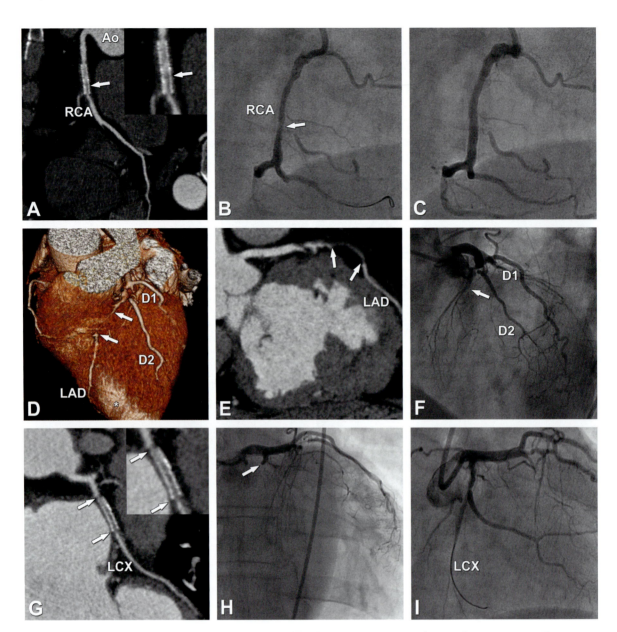

Fig. 10.33 In-stent restenosis and occlusion in a 63-year-old male patient presenting with atypical angina pectoris. The *upper row* (**Panels A–C**) shows the results for the right coronary artery (RCA), the *middle row* (**Panels D–F**) for the left anterior descending coronary artery (LAD), and the *bottom row* (**Panels G–I**) for the left circumflex coronary artery (LCX). Because of the presence of hypodense material in the distal part of the RCA stent (*arrow* in **Panel A**, curved multiplanar reformation), CT suspected significant in-stent restenosis (see inset in **Panel A** for a magnified view). Conventional angiography was initiated and confirmed a significant in-stent restenosis in the mid-segment of the RCA (*arrow* in **Panel B**). Percutaneous coronary intervention was performed during the same angiographic session (**Panel C**). CT also showed a known occlusion of the LAD (*arrows*), as depicted here in a three-dimensional volume-rendered reconstruction (**Panel D**), and a curved multiplanar reformation along the vessel (**Panel E**), which was confirmed on conventional angiography (**Panel F**). There were intracoronary LAD collaterals via septal branches that bypassed the occlusion, as seen on CT (**Panels D** and **E**). The LAD occlusion had resulted in apical infarction causing wall thinning (*asterisk* in **Panel D**). The second stent in the proximal left circumflex coronary artery (LCX) was filled with hypodense material (*arrows* in **Panel G**, curved multiplanar reformation), and based on coronary CT, occlusion of this stent was suspected (see inset in **Panel G** for a magnified view). Conventional angiography also confirmed stent occlusion in the proximal LCX (*arrow* in **Panel H**), and the stent was percutaneously recanalized in the same angiographic session (**Panel I**). *D1* first diagonal branch (segment 9); *D2* second diagonal branch (segment 10)

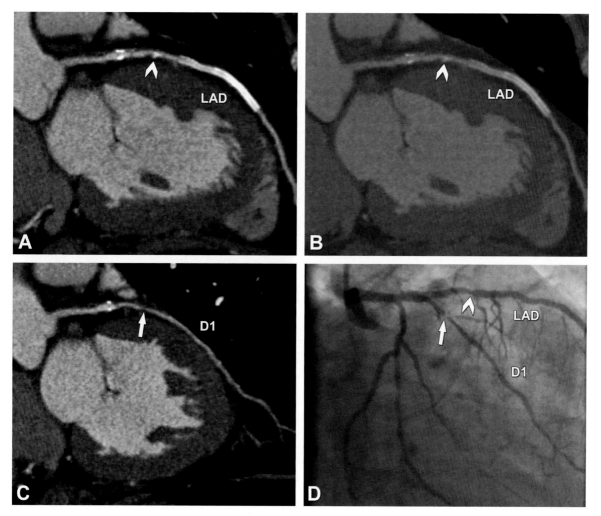

Fig. 10.34 Importance of stent kernels for evaluation of coronary stents. This 53-year-old male patient presenting with typical angina pectoris had a history of stenting of the left anterior descending coronary artery (LAD), with two 2.5-mm diameter stents. Curved multiplanar reformation based on standard reconstruction kernel for coronary arteries did not allow reliable assessment of the stent lumen (**Panel A**). Use of stent kernels, however, showed no sign of in-stent restenosis (**Panel B**). Also, the calcified plaque (*arrowhead* in **Panels A** and **B**) was easier to assess using a stent kernel, and significant luminal diameter reduction resulting from this plaque was excluded (**Panel B**). However, a 90% diameter stenosis (*arrow*) of the first diagonal branch (D1), caused by a noncalcified plaque (**Panel C**), was confirmed on conventional angiography (*arrow* in **Panel D**). Conventional coronary angiography also confirmed that the calcified plaque in the mid-LAD caused only a nonsignificant reduction in diameter (*arrowhead* in **Panel D**)

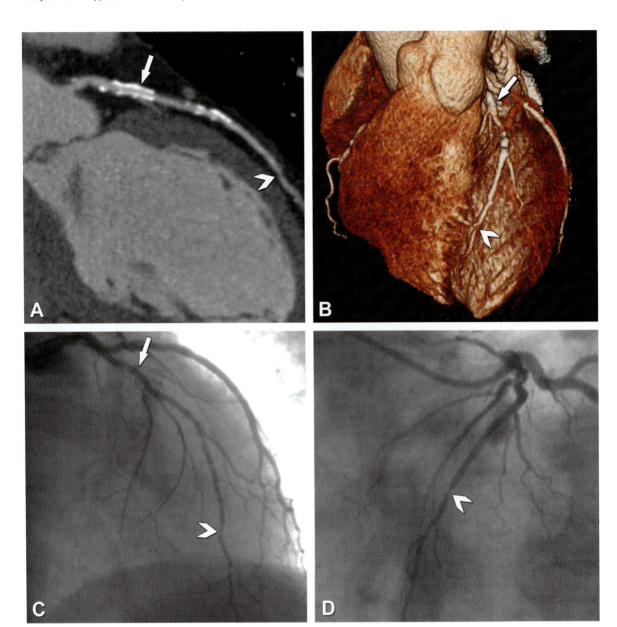

Fig. 10.35 Exclusion of significant in-stent restenosis in the left anterior descending coronary artery in a 70-year-old male patient. The 3.5-mm diameter stent was unremarkable on curved multiplanar reformation of coronary CT (*arrow* in **Panel A**), but a 60% diameter stenosis resulting from a noncalcified plaque was suspected in the distal left anterior descending artery (*arrowhead* in **Panels A** and **B**). Conventional coronary angiography confirmed the patency of the stent (*arrow* in **Panel C**), but the distal stenosis was considered on quantitative analysis to represent a 40% diameter reduction (*arrowhead* in **Panels C** and **D**). This example further illustrates the fact that there is sometimes less-than-perfect agreement between CT and conventional angiography in terms of quantifying coronary artery stenoses. Such disagreements are attributable to the three-dimensional nature of CT, which is advantageous (**Fig. 10.16**) in that it allows a more accurate assessment of diameter reduction, especially in the case of bifurcation lesions; in contrast, the relevantly higher spatial resolution of conventional angiography is a pivotal advantage of this test

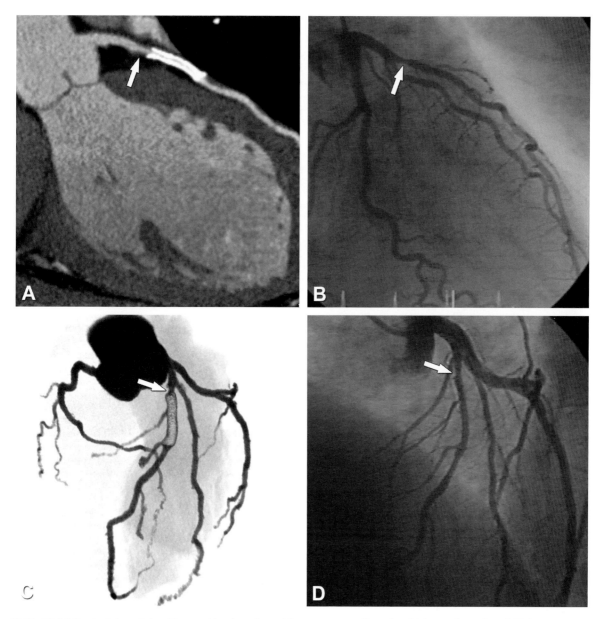

Fig. 10.36 Prestent stenosis in a 45-year-old male patient without symptoms. Curved multiplanar reformation of CT demonstrates a 30% diameter reduction in the lumen immediately proximal to the stent, resulting from a noncalcified plaque (*arrow* in **Panel A**). Significant in-stent restenosis was excluded using stent kernel curved multiplanar reformations (not shown). Conventional angiography also demonstrated the 30% prestent stenosis (*arrow* in **Panel B**). Angiographic emulation of coronary CT angiography nicely demonstrated the stenosis (*arrow* in **Panel C**), with an excellent correlation with conventional angiography (*arrow* in **Panel D**). Note that the angiographic emulation of CT has the advantage of simultaneously depicting the left and right coronary artery

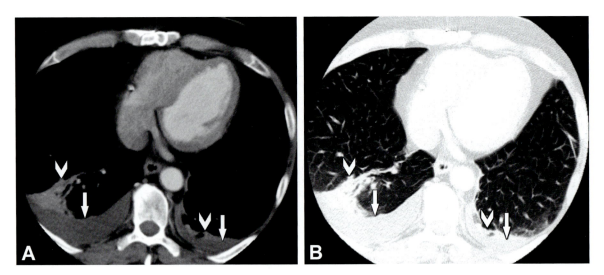

Fig. 10.37 Postoperative bilateral pleural effusion (*arrows*) in a 61-year-old male patient who underwent bypass grafting. Results are shown on large fields of view with soft tissue (**Panel A**) and lung window-level settings (**Panel B**). Note that the effusions cause (nonobstructive) atelectasis in both lower lobes (*arrowheads*)

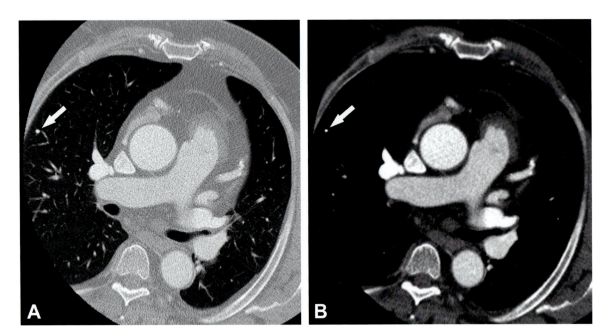

Fig. 10.38 Calcified pulmonary nodule 0.4 cm in diameter (in the size range of 0.3–0.5 cm, lesions are called "ditzels") in the middle lobe (*arrow* in **Panels A** and **B**) in a 61-year-old male patient without known malignancy. The appearance is characteristic for calcified granuloma that is most likely caused by a prior infection (e.g., tuberculosis, histoplasmosis)

10.6 · Noncardiac Findings

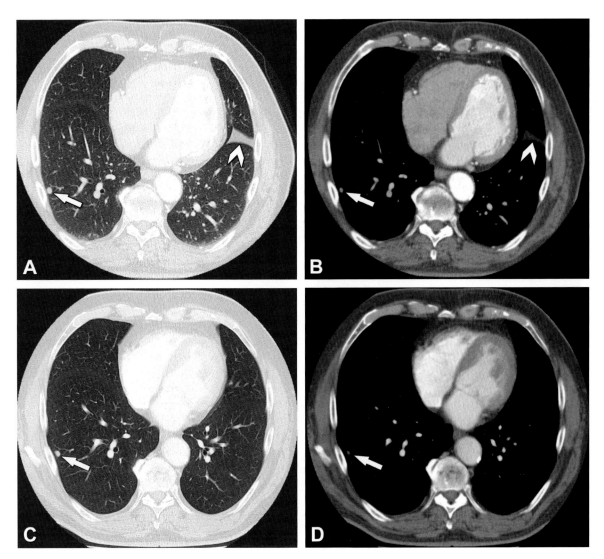

Fig. 10.39 A solitary pulmonary nodule (0.7 cm) in the right lower lobe (*arrow* in **Panels A** and **B**) that is well-circumscribed, predominantly solid, and does not contain any calcifications. There is also an effusion in the left oblique fissure (*arrowhead* in **Panels A** and **B**) Guideline-based 6-month follow-up (according to MacMahon et al. Radiology 2005) standard chest CT was performed, which showed a minor decrease in size and ruled out potential malignancy (*arrow* in **Panels C** and **D**). Differential diagnoses for such nodules include benign infectious lesions, atypical adenomatous hyperplasia, metastases, and lung cancer. Follow-up CT scans can serve to differentiate benign and malignant pulmonary nodules in indeterminate cases

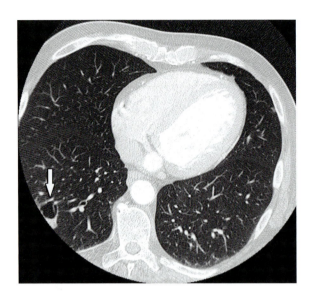

Fig. 10.40 Cavernous lung lesion in the right lower lobe (*arrow*) in a 56-year-old male patient presenting with atypical angina pectoris, who was referred to rule out coronary artery stenoses. There were no significant coronary stenoses, and the nodule with a thin-walled cavity was found on the large fields of view only and was suspected to be due to tuberculosis. Transthoracic biopsy, however, was initiated and revealed a lung carcinoma. Note that because a medium-size scan field of view (320 mm) was chosen for acquisition (to allow using a small focus spot), the reconstruction field of view cannot be larger than 320 mm, and thus the carcinoma is only partially visible

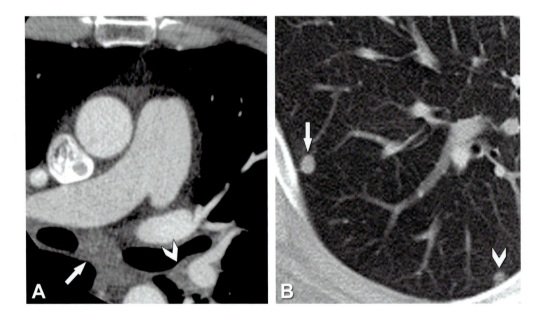

Fig. 10.41 Infracarinal 2 × 1.5 cm mediastinal lymph node (*arrow*) and peribronchial thickening (*arrowhead* in **Panel A**) in a 48-year-old male patient. Pulmonary nodules (*arrow*) and pleural-based opacities were also visible (*arrowhead* in **Panel B**). The final diagnosis was pulmonary sarcoidosis. Common differential diagnoses of mediastinal lymph nodes include lymph node metastases, lymphoma, sarcoidosis, amyloidosis, and silicosis

10.6 · Noncardiac Findings

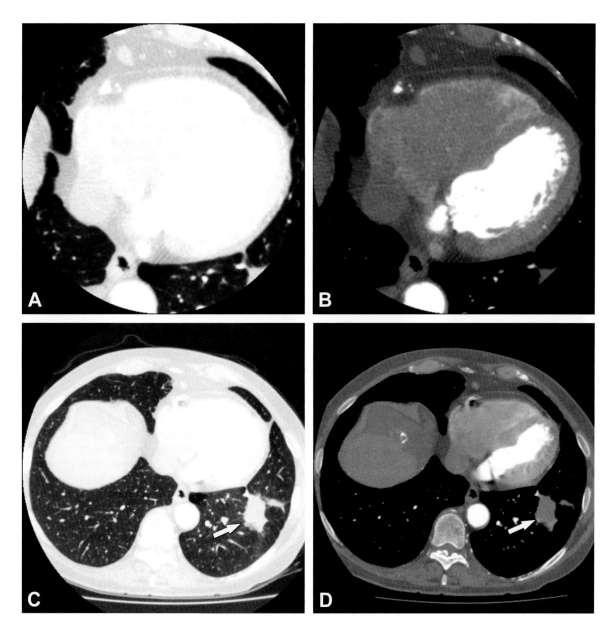

Fig. 10.42 Incidental finding of a lung carcinoma in the left lower lobe not recognized on dedicated small reconstruction fields of view for coronary artery evaluation (**Panels A** and **B**) but visible on the large fields of view with a 320 mm size (*arrow* in **Panels C** and **D**) The *left column* represents lung window-level settings, and the *right column* soft tissue window-level settings. The irregular 2.5 cm mass in the left lower lobe was spiculated and had pleural tails (**Panels C** and **D**), highly suspicious of malignancy. Both bronchoalveolar lavage and transbronchial biopsies were negative (no malignant cells found). However, transthoracic CT-guided lung biopsy resulted in a diagnosis of nonsmall cell lung carcinoma. A positron-emission tomography scan showed no signs of metastasis, and the patient underwent lobectomy of the left lower lobe with partial lingula resection. The final diagnosis was adenocarcinoma, with spread into the lingula and visceral pleura. There were free margins after resection, and no peribronchial metastases (complete resection of a pT2N0M0 tumor). This case underlines how important it is to always reconstruct the lungs on large fields so as to avoid overlooking any pathology. Coronary CT angiography was performed in this 72-year-old female patient before renal transplantation for renal failure resulting from polycystic kidney disease. Note the partially imaged liver cyst with calcification in association with polycystic kidney disease. Images courtesy of L. Kroft

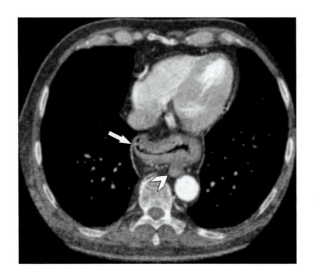

Fig. 10.43 Large hiatal hernia in an 82-year-old male patient (*arrow*). Such hernias can cause chest pain mimicking angina pectroris, and proton pump inhibitors may reduce the symptoms of reflux. The displaced esophagus is located posteriorly (*arrowhead*) to this "upside-down" stomach

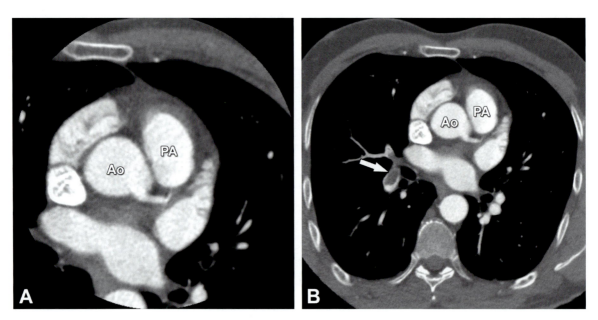

Fig. 10.44 Unexpected pulmonary embolism in a 39-year-old male patient that was not seen on dedicated small reconstruction fields of view for coronary artery evaluation (**Panel A**) but was visible on the large fields of view with 320-mm size (*arrow* in **Panel B**). Note the filling defect in the interlobar pulmonary artery, which was only seen on large-field reconstruction (*arrow* in **Panel B**). Extensive pulmonary embolism was found in the right middle and lower lobes at maximum reconstruction fields-of-view. The patient had to be readmitted for medical treatment of this complication. Coronary CT angiography was performed for evaluation of scar tissue and/or complications after right ventricular radiofrequency ablation therapy of an arrhythmia focus. This case again demonstrates that large fields of view should always be reconstructed and evaluated. Images courtesy of L. Kroft

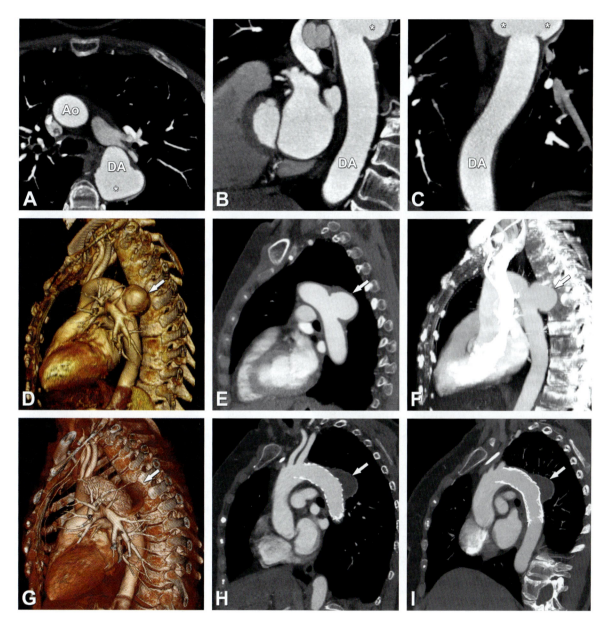

Fig. 10.45 Saccular aneurysm of the descending thoracic aorta in a 65-year-old female patient. On the most cranial slices of coronary CT angiography, a focal excentric dilatation (4.3 cm, *asterisks* in **Panels A–C**) of the descending aorta (DA) is partially visible. **Panel A** represents an axial source image, and **Panels B** and **C** represent double-oblique sagittal and coronal slices. Because of this extracardiac finding, CT angiography of the thoracic and abdominal aorta was subsequently performed. This test confirmed the focal saccular aneurysm, which did not extend to the aortic arch (*arrow* in **Panels D–F**, lateral views). Percutaneous interventional treatment with stenting was performed, and follow-up CT scans showed that the stent excluded the aneurysm well, resulting in thrombosis and exclusion from perfusion of the aneurysm (*arrow* in **Panels G–I**, lateral views). The suprarenal location and the absence of atherosclerosis in other vascular territories indicate that this was most likely a mycotic aneurysm. *Ao* aorta

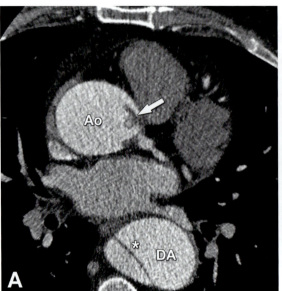
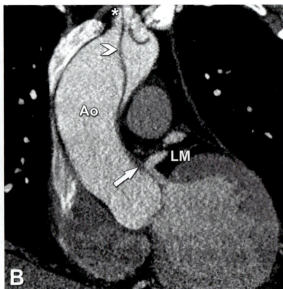
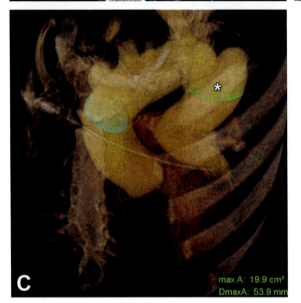

Fig. 10.46 Aortic dissection (Stanford and DeBakey type I) with obstruction of the left main coronary artery ostium and extension into the descending aorta (DA) in a 48-year-old male patient presenting with acute thoracic back pain. Axial source images (**Panel A**) and double-oblique coronal images (**Panel B**) demonstrate the dissection membrane in the ascending aorta (*arrowhead* in **Panel B**) and descending aorta (*asterisk* in **Panel A**). The dissection extends into the innominate artery (brachiocephalic trunk, *asterisk* in **Panel B**) and obstructs the left main coronary ostium (LM, *arrow* in **Panels A** and **B**). Automatic measurement of the inner diameters of the thoracic aorta was performed (**Panel C**) and revealed a maximum diameter of 5.4 cm (descending aortic aneurysm). The advantage of this comprehensive ECG-synchronized CT imaging approach is that the coronary arteries can be simultaneously evaluated. Emergency aortic repair and bypass grafting (left internal mammary artery to the left anterior descending and venous bypass graft to the left circumflex) was performed

10.6 • Noncardiac Findings

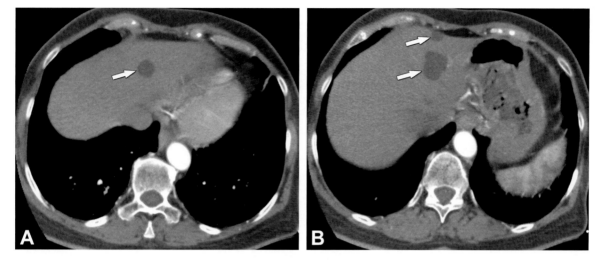

Fig. 10.47 Incidental finding of multiple (up to 2.5 cm) liver cysts (*arrows* in **Panels A** and **B**) in a 66-year-old female patient who underwent coronary CT angiography that excluded significant coronary artery stenoses. Differentiating liver cysts from low-density metastases or liver tumors can be difficult because only the purely arterial phase of liver perfusion is available with coronary CT. Thus, dedicated liver imaging, e.g., using ultrasound, is recommended whenever liver lesions that are suspicious for malignancy or not seen on prior imaging are detected

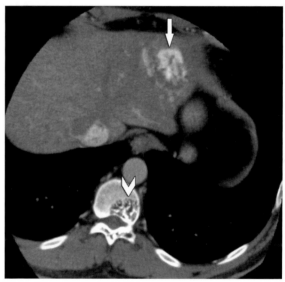

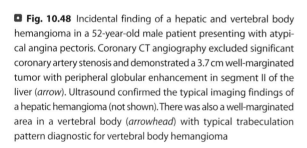

Fig. 10.48 Incidental finding of a hepatic and vertebral body hemangioma in a 52-year-old male patient presenting with atypical angina pectoris. Coronary CT angiography excluded significant coronary artery stenosis and demonstrated a 3.7 cm well-marginated tumor with peripheral globular enhancement in segment II of the liver (*arrow*). Ultrasound confirmed the typical imaging findings of a hepatic hemangioma (not shown). There was also a well-marginated area in a vertebral body (*arrowhead*) with typical trabeculation pattern diagnostic for vertebral body hemangioma

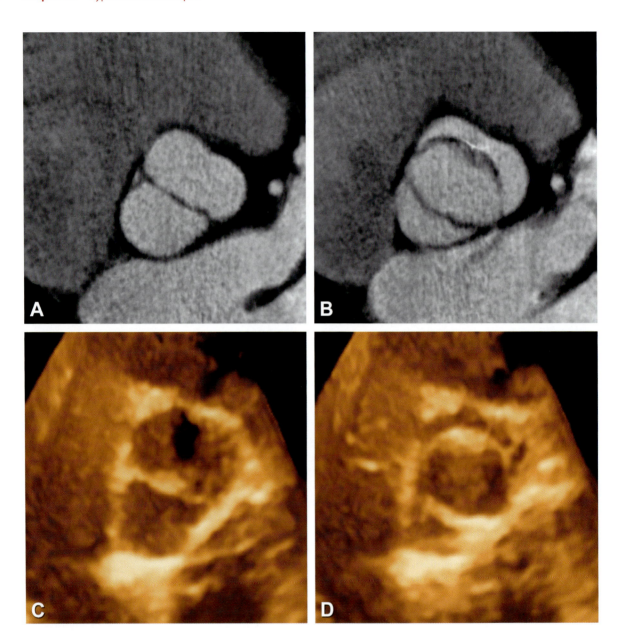

Fig. 10.49 Bicuspid aortic valve in a 48-year-old male patient. There is normal closure (**Panel A**) and opening of the aortic valve (**Panel B**) as seen with CT. CT data are shown as minimum-intensity projections. There is excellent correlation with the findings of three-dimensional transthoracic echocardiography (**Panels C** and **D**). Echocardiography images courtesy of A.C. Borges

10.7 · Extracoronary Cardiac Findings

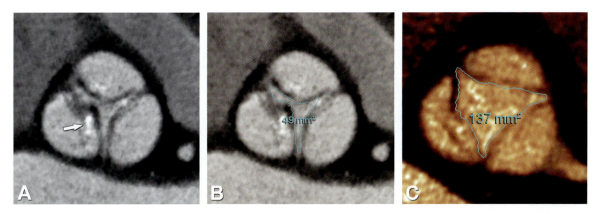

Fig. 10.50 Tricuspid aortic valve in an 83-year-old female patient with stenosis. There are moderate calcifications of the aortic cusps (*arrow* in **Panel A**) that lead to severe (<1.0 cm²) stenosis of the valve during systole (**Panel A**). Caliper measurement of the aortic valve area during systole (**Panel B**) shows a valve area of 0.49 cm². After surgical replacement of the valve, there is marked increase in the systolic aortic valve area (**Panel C**). Mild and moderate aortic valve stenoses are represented by aortic valve areas of >1.5 cm² and 1.0–1.5 cm², respectively. CT data are shown as minimum-intensity projections

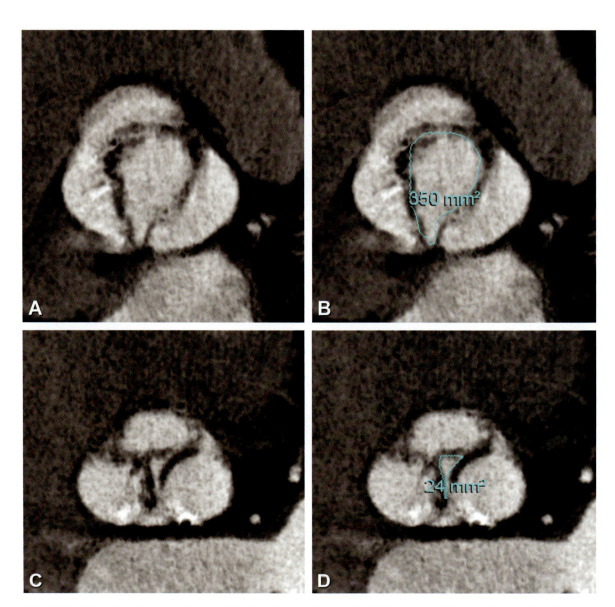

Fig. 10.51 Tricuspid aortic valve with regurgitation in a 48-year-old male patient. **Panels A** and **B** show results of systole with normal opening of the valve cusps, while **Panels C** and **D** show the aortic regurgitation area during diastole (0.24 cm²). The right column shows the caliper measurements of the aortic valve area. CT data are shown as minimum-intensity projections

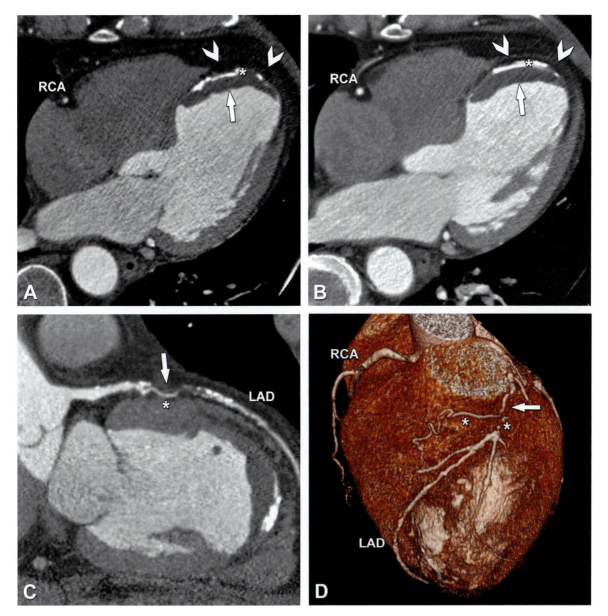

Fig. 10.52 Left ventricular apical aneurysm with thrombus in a 79-year-old male patient with a history of anterior myocardial infarction 19 years ago, who had suspected thrombus on transthoracic echocardiography. There is a left ventricular crescent-filling defect (*arrow* in **Panel A**), representing an apical thrombus. The thrombus is due to stasis of blood in the akinetic apical aneurysm resulting from chronic myocardial infarction. The myocardial infarct has resulted in myocardial calcification (*asterisk* in **Panel A**) and fatty degeneration (*arrowheads* in **Panel A**). The fatty changes in the myocardium are seen as densities similar to those of the pericardial fat. **Panel A** is a four-chamber view of the left ventricle obtained with a 0.5 mm slice thickness. For comparison, the findings are also shown as a 5 mm thin-slab maximum-intensity projection in the four-chamber view (**Panel B**) The myocardial infarction was the result of an occlusion of the left anterior descending coronary artery (LAD, *arrow* in **Panels C** and **D**). Left-to-left collaterals (*asterisks* in **Panels C** and **D**) bypass the occlusion. Nevertheless, a large infarction with an apical aneurysm and thrombus formation eventually occurred in this patient. *RCA* right coronary artery

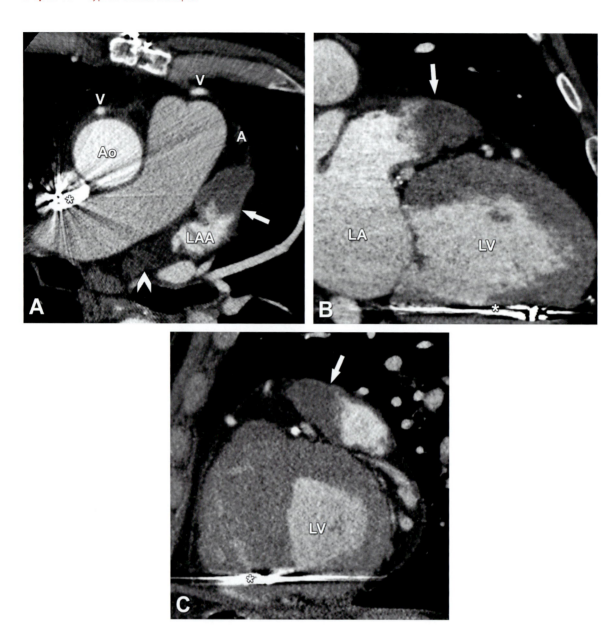

Fig. 10.53 Left atrial thrombus in a 65-year-old male patient presenting 6 months after arterial (A) and venous (V) bypass grafting. The thrombus (*arrow*) is seen in the left atrial appendage (LAA) on axial (**Panel A**), coronal (**Panel B**), and sagittal images (**Panel C**). The patient also has a cardiac defibrillator (*asterisk* in **Panels A–C**). The left pulmonic pericardial recess (*arrowhead*) is seen in **Panel A** and can be differentiated from thrombotic material because it has lower density. Adding a late phase (2 min after contrast agent injection) increases confidence in the use of cardiac CT in the diagnosis of atrial thrombi. *Ao* aorta; *LA* left atrium; *LV* left ventricle

10.7 · Extracoronary Cardiac Findings

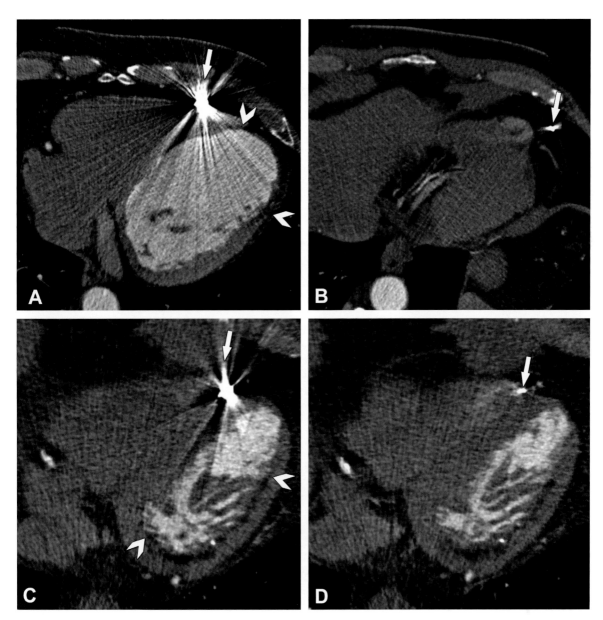

Fig. 10.54 Right ventricular lead perforation of an automated implantable cardioverter defibrillator in a 57-year-old male patient who had pacemaker dysfunction on testing. In **Panel A**, the lead is still in the right ventricle (*arrow*), and an apical infarction (*arrowheads*) is visible. A few slices further caudally, the tip of the lead can be seen penetrating into the pericardial cavity (*arrow* in **Panel B**) For comparison, the same anatomical regions are shown in a different 67-year-old male patient presenting with typical angina pectoris (**Panels C** and **D**). This patient has an inferolateral myocardial infarction (*arrowheads* in **Panel C**), and the tip of the lead is located within the right ventricle (*arrow* in **Panel D**)

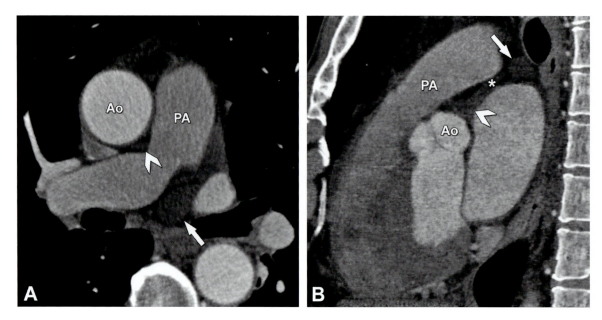

Fig. 10.55 Pericardial recesses and sinuses need to be differentiated from effusions, lymph nodes, and dissections. **Panels A** and **B** show an example of a left pulmonic pericardial recess (*arrow*) in the groove inferior to the left pulmonary artery (PA). This recess commonly communicates (*asterisk* in **Panel B**) with the transverse pericardial sinus (*arrowhead* in **Panel B**), which is located posterior to the ascending aorta (Ao). Also communicating with the transverse sinus is the superior aortic recess (*arrowhead* in **Panel A**). The posterior pericardial recess (not shown) is also sometimes seen and is located posterior to the right pulmonary artery as part of the oblique pericardial sinus. The typical location and CT appearance (density of water, well-marginated, tapered configuration) allow pericardial recesses to be distinguished from mediastinal lymphadenopathy, pericardial effusions, and aortic dissection

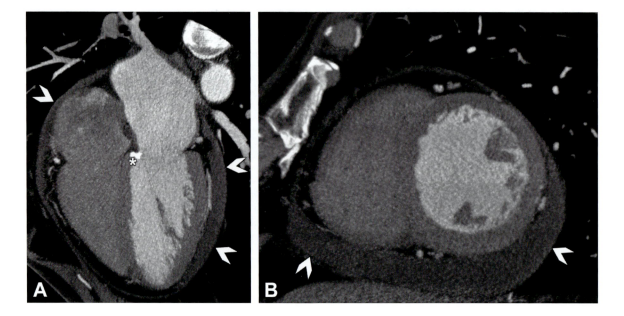

Fig. 10.56 Pericardial effusion (with a 2 cm posterior width) in a 61-year-old male patient 6 months after coronary artery stenting. Both the four-chamber view (**Panel A**) and the cardiac short-axis view (**Panel B**) show the large pericardial effusion (*arrowheads*). There is a small mitral valve annulus calcification (*asterisk* in **Panel A**), another noncoronary cardiac finding. CT data are shown as maximum-intensity projections

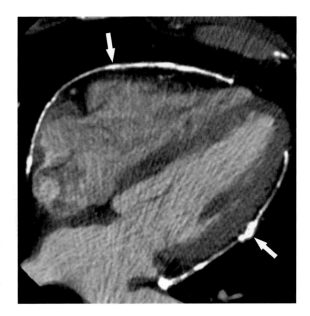

Fig. 10.57 Circumferential calcification of the pericardium (*arrows*) in a four-chamber view. Such calcifications typically cause constrictive pericarditis, which can be associated with elevated right cardiac pressures, dyspnea, exercise intolerance, and even ascites. Most pericardial calcifications have an infectious etiology (e.g., tuberculosis, histoplasmosis)

Results of Clinical Studies

M. Dewey

11.1 Coronary Arteries..................... 181
11.2 Coronary Artery Bypasses 181
11.3 Coronary Artery Stents............... 181
11.4 Cardiac Function 181

> **Abstract**
>
> This chapter summarizes the diagnostic performance of coronary CT angiography.

11.1 Coronary Arteries

Noninvasive coronary angiography using multislice CT as a means of ruling out significant stenoses in patients with low-to-intermediate likelihood of disease is the foremost clinical application of this test. Numerous single and multicenter studies have addressed the diagnostic performance of CT in detecting stenoses of the native coronary vessels, and we have summarized the results in terms of per-patient sensitivity and specificity in **Fig. 11.1**. Please note that the negative predictive value of CT is 95% in this analysis (data not shown in the figure) and represents the major advantage of this test (Chap. 5).

11.2 Coronary Artery Bypasses

Assessing coronary arterial and venous bypass grafts is an important application of CT in some patients (e.g., patients with recurrent chest pain and equivocal stress results). Numerous single-center studies have addressed the diagnostic performance of CT in coronary artery bypass grafts, and we have summarized the results as per-graft sensitivity and specificity in **Figs. 11.2** and **11.3**.

11.3 Coronary Artery Stents

The successful detection of coronary artery stent stenoses with CT is limited when compared with assessment of the native vessels using current technology. Sufficient image quality and accuracy are, in general, achieved only for large stents (at least 3.5-mm diameter). In the case of smaller stents, only about 50% of cases are evaluable. Numerous single-center studies and one multicenter study have addressed the diagnostic performance of CT in detecting in-stent restenoses, and we have summarized the results as per-stent sensitivity and specificity in **Fig. 11.4**. Please note that the positive predictive value is only 70% in this analysis (data not shown in the figure), a major limitation of CT for coronary stent evaluation.

11.4 Cardiac Function

Global and regional cardiac function can easily be assessed using the same data that have been acquired for coronary CT angiography. Because it has considerable influence on patient management (Chap. 9), left ventricular function should be evaluated in all patients undergoing cardiac CT. We have summarized the accuracy of CT in determining left ventricular ejection in **Fig. 11.5**.

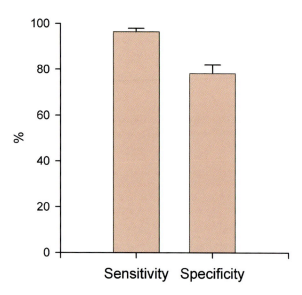

Fig. 11.1 Per-patient diagnostic performance (sensitivity, specificity, and nondiagnostic rate) of coronary CT angiography in native coronary vessels, when compared with conventional coronary angiography as the reference (gold) standard. Results were obtained using all published studies on this topic. Error bars represent 95% confidence intervals. Please note that because this figure represents per-patient results, direct comparison with the following figures (per-graft and per-stent results) is not possible

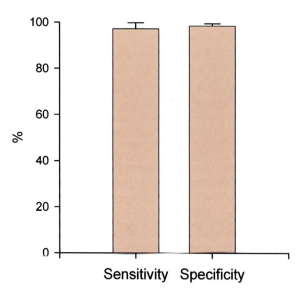

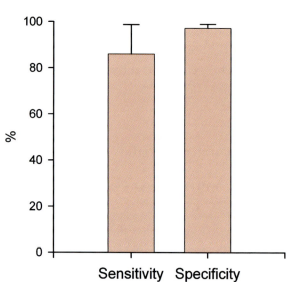

Fig. 11.2 Per-graft diagnostic performance (sensitivity, specificity) of coronary CT angiography in detecting coronary artery bypass graft occlusion, when compared with conventional coronary angiography as the reference (gold) standard. Results were obtained using all published studies on this topic. Error bars represent 95% confidence intervals

Fig. 11.3 Per-graft diagnostic performance (sensitivity, specificity) of coronary CT angiography in detecting coronary artery bypass graft stenosis, when compared with conventional coronary angiography as the reference (gold) standard. Results were obtained using all published studies on this topic. Error bars represent 95% confidence intervals

11.4 · Cardiac Function

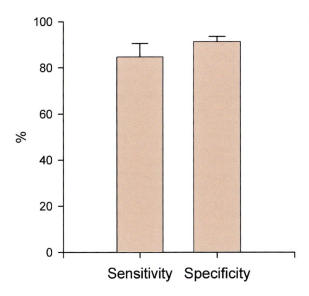

Fig. 11.4 Diagnostic performance (sensitivity and specificity) of coronary CT angiography in detecting coronary artery in-stent restenoses, when compared with conventional coronary angiography as the reference (gold) standard. Results were obtained using all published studies on this topic. Please note that patients with overall non-assessable image quality had to be excluded from this summary, as most studies did not provide detailed information about how many stents were present in these patients. Moreover, in patients with overall acceptable image quality, the per-stent nondiagnostic rate was 15%. Error bars represent 95% confidence intervals

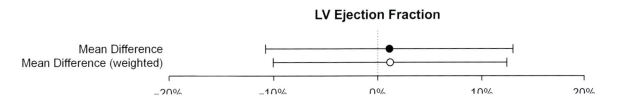

Fig. 11.5 Bland-Altman analysis of the accuracy of CT in determining left ventricular ejection fraction, vs. magnetic resonance imaging as the reference standard. Results are shown as unweighted and weighted (according to study size) mean values and limits of agreement (±95% confidence intervals). The limits of agreement indicate the expected maximum difference between CT and the reference standard and are approximately ±12%. The agreement between cineventriculography and echocardiography and the reference standard is significantly lower than that of CT, as shown in head-to-head comparisons. There is a slight underestimation of the ejection fraction by CT (as identified by the mean of approximately +2%)

Outlook

M. Dewey

12.1	Technical Developments	185
12.1.1	Cylindrical CT (Wide-Area Detector CT)	185
12.1.2	Multisource Scanning	186
12.1.3	Better Temporal Resolution	186
12.1.4	Better Spatial Resolution	187
12.2	Clinical Developments	187
12.2.1	Coronary Stent Imaging	187
12.2.2	Acute Chest Pain	188
12.2.3	Coronary Plaque Quantification and Characterization	188
12.2.4	High-Risk Patients	188

Abstract

This chapter discusses anticipated technical and clinical developments with regard to CT.

12.1 Technical Developments

Technical developments expected in the near future are summarized in **List 12.1**.

List 12.1. The foremost upcoming technical developments

1. Cylindrical CT (wide-area detector) covering the entire heart in one rotation
2. Multisource CT, potentially further improving temporal resolution
3. Further reduction in gantry rotation times
4. Further reduction in slice collimation

12.1.1 Cylindrical CT (Wide-Area Detector CT)

The recently approved and released 320-slice CT scanners (with wide-area detectors), which image the body in a cylindrical fashion ("cylindrical CT," **Fig. 12.1**, are able to scan the entire heart during a single rotation without any table movement (**Fig. 12.2**). Thus, this technology will greatly reduce the scan time for coronary angiography from 8 to 10 s for 64-slice CT to less than 1 s in patients with low heart rates. This improvement significantly reduces the likelihood of both ECG and breathing-related motion artifacts and thus improves image quality. Moreover, the prospective acquisitions with cylindrical CT that cover the entire heart without over-sampling and over-ranging will reduce the effective dose by a factor of 3–5 to an average of less than 5 mSv for coronary angiography in patients with low and stable heart rates. These improvements have great potential for further promoting the widespread clinical application of coronary CT angiography.

The amount of contrast agent required is further reduced with cylindrical wide-area detector CT. However, a drawback of the new scanner is that the increased width of the detector (by a factor of 5) will increase scattered radiation, and therefore image noise. To compensate for this scatter, the tube current may have to be slightly increased from that of 64-slice CT (to about 400 mA). Nevertheless, image quality will be improved with cylindrical CT, and radiation exposure will be significantly reduced. Another advantage of this new type of CT scanner is that a fourth dimension, time, is added to the scanning, making it possible to assess myocardial perfusion and coronary blood flow ("dynamic volume CT"). In this way, CT might to some extent be able to replace conventional approaches involving myocardial perfusion imaging, while providing information on coronary stenoses and plaques.

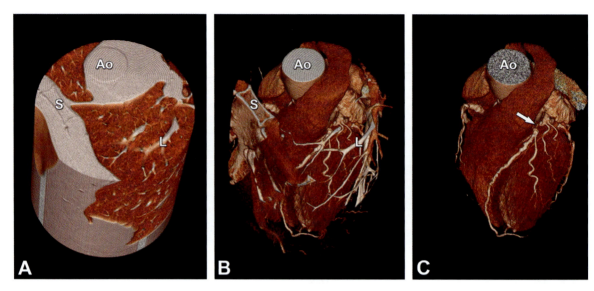

Fig. 12.1 Cardiac imaging with cylindrical CT using 320 simultaneous detector rows shows the cylindrical appearance of the volume, which was prospectively scanned within a single heart beat (**Panel A**). Thus, this new CT technique is also referred to as "cylindrical wide-area detector CT." After changing the window-level settings of this three-dimensional reconstruction, the lung veins (*L*) become evaluable (**Panel B**). Using automatic segmentation tools (**Panel C**) the heart and coronary vessels are isolated, and a significant stenosis becomes visible in the left anterior descending coronary artery (*arrow*). *Ao* aorta; *S* sternum

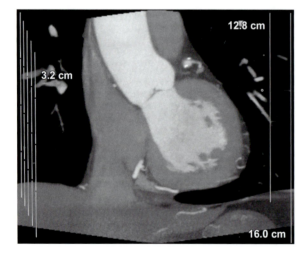

Fig. 12.2 Scanning of the entire heart in one rotation with cylindrical CT using 320-slice technology and a coverage of 16.0 cm (superimposed on a coronal maximum-intensity projection of the left ventricle and aorta), compared with conventional coverage using 64-slice CT with 3.2-cm detector width (left side of image, based on a pitch of 0.2). Please note that the angle of the X-ray beam using 320 simultaneous detector rows is 15°. Thus, the volume acquired with a single X-ray shot looks like a cylinder bounded by two circular cones (**Fig. 12.1**)

12.1.2 Multisource Scanning

Dual-source CT has been available for some time now and has been of great value in improving temporal resolution and reducing the dependency on heart rate. It is expected that further technical developments will lead to the availability of clinical multisource CT scanners, which could further reduce the length of the image reconstruction windows within the RR interval. In this way, coronary CT angiography could become fully independent of heart rate. However, scattered radiation also increases when more X-ray tubes are used.

A limitation of the current dual-source CT technology is its inability to reduce the overall scanning time or the likelihood of ECG and breathing-related artifacts. It is, therefore, more than likely that the concepts of cylindrical and multisource CT will eventually be merged within a single CT scanner, making the advantages of both approaches available for patient care.

12.1.3 Better Temporal Resolution

Further reducing the gantry rotation time (to below the currently achieved 270–350 ms) is an obvious approach to improving temporal resolution and reducing heart rate dependency. However, our ability to shorten the rotation time is limited by the dramatic increase in centrifugal forces that occurs as the rotation time is reduced. For instance, at a 400-ms rotation time, the relative centrifugal force is 18–20 g, which already requires considerable centripetal force to counteract. However, at 200 ms (equal to an image acquisition window of 100 ms with halfscan reconstruction), the relative centrifugal forces rise to 74–80 g because they are equal to the square of the velocity. New technologies such as an air-bearing CT gantry might alleviate this problem and make it feasible to reduce the rotation time to 200 ms or even shorter. However, it is not very likely that a reduction in the rotation time alone will be pursued as a strategy for further improving temporal resolution. Instead, it is much more likely that the three concepts of (1) multisource scanning, (2) adaptive multisegment reconstruction, and (3) shortening the gantry rotation time will be developed further and combined in some fashion to improve temporal resolution.

12.1.4 Better Spatial Resolution

The current slice collimation of coronary CT angiography (between 0.5 and 0.75 mm) limits its application to small structures such as coronary plaque and its internal makeup. Thus, thinner slice collimation and smaller cell width in the channel direction (e.g., of 0.2–0.3 mm) have the potential to improve the assessment of plaques and stents and facilitate the quantification of stenoses by coronary CT angiography (**Fig. 12.3**). However, reducing the slice collimation by a factor of 2 requires the radiation exposure to be increased by a factor of 2 (if the same detector technology is used) to keep the image quality constant. Thus, improvements in spatial resolution are not easily achieved using the current technology, and further developments (e.g., detector material) are necessary for clinical applications if one does not wish to increase radiation exposure again.

12.2 Clinical Developments

The expected upcoming clinical developments are summarized in **List 12.2**.

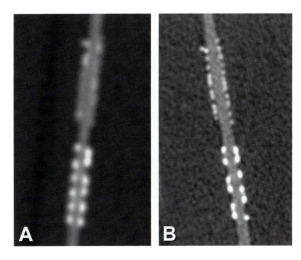

Fig. 12.3 Advantages of high-resolution CT with a ~0.3-mm slice thickness for coronary stent imaging. Multiplanar reformations along a coronary stent with 2.5-mm inner diameter (in a phantom) obtained using 0.625-mm slice collimation and cell width (**Panel A**), and high-resolution CT with 0.3-mm slice collimation and cell width using a 0.3 × 0.3-mm focus size tube (**Panel B**). The opacified lumen within the small stent is more clearly seen, with fewer blooming artifacts, using the thinner slice collimation. Images courtesy of Sachio Kuribayashi. Department of Radiology, Keio University School of Medicine

List 12.2. The foremost upcoming clinical developments

1. Reliable coronary artery stent imaging
2. Use of CT in patients presenting to the ER with acute chest pain
3. Imaging and follow-up of coronary plaques after medical interventions
4. Application of CT to asymptomatic high-risk patients

12.2.1 Coronary Stent Imaging

The technical innovations described above may make possible the reliable assessment of coronary artery stents for the presence of restenoses. For this purpose, it will be instrumental to add the fourth dimension to our analysis and to reduce motion artifacts that are related to ECG irregularities or patients' limited breath-hold capacity. Also, better spatially localized and temporally resolved quantitative measurements of the inner diameter of coronary stents will be pivotal to our efforts to broaden the clinical use of CT and extend it to the follow-up of patients who have undergone percutaneous coronary stent placement.

12.2.2 Acute Chest Pain

As is necessary for new medications, diagnostic tests should be subjected to rigorous clinical and scientific analysis, ideally in large-scale randomized trials that most accurately reflect the clinical situation and analyze true outcomes. If such studies can demonstrate the clinical utility of CT in patients presenting to the ER with acute chest pain, it is conceivable that clinical indications will be extended to these patients as well. However, a prerequisite for the wider use of coronary CT angiography is that this test can reduce hard cardiovascular events and/or complications while also being more cost-effective than conventional diagnostic approaches. It is also important to show that acute patients with a negative coronary CT angiography will have a very low long-term event rate.

12.2.3 Coronary Plaque Quantification and Characterization

One of the greatest potential advantages of coronary CT angiography is its ability to noninvasively determine the volume, characteristics, and composition of coronary artery plaques. Since most acute coronary events arise from plaques that cause only a minimal percent stenosis, it is of importance to identify plaque characteristics that are unambiguously associated with a higher risk in individual patients and would be expected to trigger intense medical treatment and preventive measures. However, such characteristics have not yet been identified. With the use of combined positron-emission tomography/CT scanners, it might be possible to identify culprit coronary plaques with increased inflammation.

Although it competes with intravascular ultrasound, CT is also a potential candidate for following up coronary artery plaques after initiation of certain medical therapies. Thus, if further large studies demonstrate its clinical validity and measuring accuracy, coronary CT angiography could become the foremost diagnostic surrogate parameter and test for analyzing the outcome of new drugs in terms of regression of coronary plaques.

12.2.4 High-Risk Patients

Since 50% of men and 64% of women who die suddenly of coronary heart disease were previously asymptomatic, it is obvious that an ongoing search is necessary to identify parameters that reliably predict such coronary events. The identification of coronary plaques and stenoses in these patients might help optimize further treatment. However, it must be borne in mind that no evidence exists that revascularization of coronary stenoses in asymptomatic patients improves outcomes. Given its current high effective dose, CT is unlikely to play a relevant role in screening of high-risk patients. If a significant dose reduction is achieved by using prospectively acquired coronary CT angiography, however, the situation requires reappraisal, and the clinical usefulness of CT for this indication must be considered anew. However, here again, large-scale randomized trials that analyze hard and soft events are necessary before a final decision can be made. Until then, coronary CT angiography is clearly not indicated in asymptomatic patients for routing clinical screening.

Index

A
Accreditation, 7
American College of Cardiology (ACC), 7–9, 120
American College of Radiology (ACR), 7, 8, 124
Angina pectoris
   atypical, 28, 31–34, 138, 140, 149, 152, 154, 160, 166, 171
   typical, 31–34, 133–135, 137, 141, 143–148, 155–158, 161, 177
Angiographic emulation, 105, 110, 115, 116, 135, 144, 163
Aortic valve, 4, 57, 60, 61, 123, 124, 172–174
Arterial bypass grafts, 6, 28, 31, 49, 51, 54, 120, 129, 148, 149, 152, 176, 181, 182,
Artifacts, 3, 4, 48, 49, 53, 54, 63, 67–69, 77, 81, 82, 90, 94, 101, 102, 107, 113–119, 127, 133, 149, 151, 156, 185–187

B
Beta blocker, 3, 8, 44, 50–53, 57, 62, 71, 72, 77, 84, 116, 124
Bolus tracking, 56, 67, 68, 87–88, 95, 96
Breathing, 4, 53, 57, 70, 71, 93–95, 117, 185, 186
Breath-hold training, 44, 47, 51, 53, 56, 70–72

C
Calcified plaque, 82, 113–115, 132, 137, 138, 141, 144, 158, 161
Calcium scoring, 27, 47–48, 88, 95
Clinical indications
   appropriate, 31–35
   no, 32, 36, 38
   potential, 35–36
Collaterals, 13, 27, 138–140, 147, 157, 160, 175
Competence, 7–9
Contraindications, 8, 38, 41, 42, 44
Contrast agent
   amount, 54–56, 68, 124, 185
   concentration, 55
   injection rate, 55, 77, 96
Coronary artery
   anatomy, 11–21
   bypass grafts, 3, 6, 27–28, 31, 54, 56, 120, 129, 137, 147–155, 170, 181–182
   dominance, 13, 14, 17, 21, 108, 127, 131
   distribution, 13, 14, 129, 130
   occlusion, 13, 28, 127, 129, 138–140, 142–143, 147, 150–154, 158, 160, 175, 182
   plaques, 55, 108, 114–116, 118, 129, 132–134, 137, 138, 141, 143, 185, 188
   segments, 4, 5, 11–21, 50, 72, 92, 101, 105, 107, 108, 113, 114, 116, 127, 137, 138, 140, 141, 143, 153
   stenoses, 17, 27, 38, 48, 55, 103, 105, 107, 108, 112, 113, 115, 116, 120, 127, 132, 135–146, 149, 162, 166, 171, 181, 183, 185, 187, 188
   stenosis characteristics, 127
   stents, 35, 51, 54, 113, 129, 135, 139, 153, 155–163, 178, 181, 183, 187–188
   variants, 22
Costs, 3, 29, 31
CT
   cylindrical, 185–187
   dual-source, 3, 51, 58, 61–64, 84, 85, 186
   dynamic volume, 185
   16-slice, 1, 3–6, 27, 28
   64-slice, 3–6, 27, 28, 44, 56, 58, 84, 116, 185, 186
   320-slice, 1, 185, 186,
   wide-area detector, 185, 186
Curved multiplanar reformations, 4, 22, 50, 55, 58, 59, 63, 75, 90, 102, 103, 107–113, 114, 115, 118, 130–135, 137–138, 141, 143, 144, 147–149, 151, 154–158, 160–163

E
ECG
   electrodes, 47, 48, 67, 77, 78, 93, 94, 97,
   editing, 68, 87, 104–105, 119
   gating, prospective, 3, 49, 57, 87, 89, 94, 95, 97, 124
   gating, retrospective, 57, 73, 87–89, 95, 124
Echocardiography, 1, 27, 29, 172, 175, 183
Economic, 4, 29
Effective dose, 6, 49, 51, 54, 185, 188
Exercise
   ECG, 135, 137, 144
   testing, 137
Extracoronary cardiac findings, 129, 172–180

F

Field of view
  reconstruction, 53, 58, 61, 63, 73, 77, 79, 82, 84, 89, 96, 116, 166
  scan, 53, 57, 63, 73, 79, 84, 88, 89, 91, 96–98, 166
Function, cardiac, 4, 24, 25, 32, 35, 54, 58, 120–123, 125, 127, 181, 183

G

Gatekeeper, 28, 48
Guideline, 7, 8, 51, 120, 124, 137, 165

H

Hands-on training, 7
Hands-on workshops, 7

I

In-stent restenosis, 155, 157, 158, 160–163
Interpretation, 1, 7, 8, 49, 113, 116, 119, 124, 127
Intravascular ultrasound, 114, 141, 145, 188

L

Learning curve, 7
Left internal mammary artery, 6, 54, 147–149, 151, 152, 154, 170

M

Magnetic resonance imaging (MRI), 1, 9, 27–29, 32, 35–36, 38, 41, 123, 183
Maximum-intensity projections, 13, 17, 19, 21, 49, 84, 103, 105, 108, 111, 114, 115, 134–135, 138, 140, 144–145, 147, 153, 175, 186
Medicare, 4
Mitral valve, 19, 21, 24, 28, 123–124, 178
Motion map, 64, 101–102
Multisegment reconstruction, 3, 51, 58, 62–63, 73, 92, 116, 187
Myocardial bridging, 17, 22, 103
Myocardial segments, 15, 24–25, 123

N

Negative predictive value, 27–28, 31, 35–36, 38, 181
Nitroglycerin, 8, 44, 49, 50, 70, 77, 124
Noncalcified plaque, 8, 113–114, 118, 132–134, 137–138, 140–141, 143, 145, 147, 155, 161–163
Noncardiac findings, 9, 129, 164–171

P

Patient
  education, 41
  information sheet, 41, 42
  positioning, 48, 49
  preparation, 1, 7, 41–45, 67, 77, 87, 93
  referral, 38
  referral form, 38
Pericardial recesses, 178
Pericardial sinus, 178
Performing coronary CT, 35
Positive predictive value, 28, 31–32, 35, 181
Preoxygenation, 6, 44, 53
Pre-test likelihood, 28, 29, 31, 32, 38, 48, 130
Pseudostenosis, 111, 119
Purchase, 3–4

Q

Quantification, coronary stenoses, 107, 187

R

Radiation exposure, 6, 27, 29, 32, 38, 41, 44, 47, 48, 53, 67, 70, 77, 80, 91, 95, 185, 187
Reading, 5, 31, 48, 57, 94, 101–123
Reconstruction increment, 58
Reconstruction phase, 57, 58, 61, 63, 99, 127
Reconstructions, available, 105
Remodeling index, 133–134
Reporting, 8, 25, 122, 124–127
Requirements, 3, 5–9, 73
Requirements, Technical, 3
Right internal mammary artery, 51, 148

S

Saline flush, 54, 67, 68, 77
Scan range, 47, 49, 51–54, 67
Scanning parameters, 52–54, 56, 67, 71, 72, 89, 96, 97
Screening, 28, 29, 38, 188
Single-photon emission computed tomography (SPECT), 133, 138, 140
Sinus of Valsalva, 11, 17, 22, 23
Slice collimation, 3, 47, 58, 59, 116, 187
Slice thickness, 17, 19, 57–58, 73–74, 89, 91, 175, 187
Spatial Resolution, 48, 51, 53, 57, 58, 60–61, 69, 77, 116, 158, 162, 187

T

Temporal Resolution, 3, 11, 53, 58–64, 84, 92, 116, 186–187
Test bolus, 56, 67, 68, 77–79, 95, 96
Thrombus
  left atrial, 176
  left ventricular, 175
Tube current, 54–55, 68, 72, 87, 89, 185
  modulation, 54

V

Valsava maneuver, 44, 54, 117
Venous bypass grafts, 51, 56, 129, 150–156, 181
Volume-rendering, 92, 105, 107, 115–116

W

Window-level settings, 107, 113, 114, 117, 141, 164, 167, 186